Reverse Gut Diseases Naturally is dedicated to all of my past, present and future patients. Because of my work with you, I continue to learn and expand my own knowledge in accordance to your needs. Sharing information and helping one person at a time is how we continue to be of service to each other.

This book is also dedicated to: all the practitioners and scientists who have worked so hard to give consumers the right to choose their own form of health care and wellness; to the retailers and manufacturers of natural health products, for providing people the choice of complementary medicine; and lastly, to the many authors discussing gut dysbiosis disorders, for their work in enlightening and assisting the general public.

CONTENTS

Acknowledgements   xi

Foreword by Ellen Tart-Jensen, Ph.D., D.Sc. C.C.I.I.   xiii

Preface   xvii

CHAPTER ONE

Common Denominators for Chronic Digestive Complaints   1

Bowel Disorders are Related to Other Disease Complaints   1

Assessing the Problems of Intestinal Health   2

The Healing Power of Plants   3

Leaky Gut Triggers Auto-Immune Response   3

The Diet's Crucial Influence   4

The Origin of Crohn's and Colitis Complaints   5

Medications Increase Nutritional Requirements   7

CHAPTER TWO

Empowering the Body to Heal   9

The Goal of the Digestive Process   9

Recommended Diet for Healthy Digestion   10

Thyroid and Adrenal Gland Support   11

Thyroid Gland   11

How Does the Thyroid Gland Affect My Health?   12

The TSH Test: How Accurate is It?   13

Adrenal Stress Inhibits Conversion of T4 to T3   15

A Closer Look at Thyroid Testing   15

Relationship between FT4, FT3, RT3 and TSH   15

Gluten Impacts the Thyroid Gland   17

How Do I Care for My Thyroid?   18

Nutrition for Disorders of the Thyroid Gland   18

Adrenal Glands   20

Adrenal Gland Dysfunction   21

Can the Adrenal Glands Contribute to Weight Gain?   22

What Nutrients Assist the Adrenal Glands?   23

Nutritional Recommendations for Adrenal Glands   23

CHAPTER THREE

Past, Present and Future Direction of Bowel Disorders   25

History of Inflammatory Bowel Disorders (IBD)   25

Medications Prescribed for Gastrointestinal Complaints   28

Diarrhea Overview   32

Constipation Overview   32

Diverticulosis and Diverticulitis Overview   34

Irritable Bowel Syndrome (IBS) Overview   36

Celiac Disease Overview   38

Crohn's Disease/Ulcerative Colitis (Pancolitis) Overview   40

CHAPTER FOUR

Holistic Approach for Certain Intestinal Disease Complications   43

About Type 'A' Crohn's Disease and Chronic Crohn's Disease Patients   43

Leaky Gut Syndrome is Associated with Most Gut Dysbiosis   44

Nutritional Recommendations   45

Lab Tests for Leaky Gut   46

Abscesses and Fistulas   47

Nutrition Suggestions   47

Herbal Remedies   48

Retention Enemas   50

Homeopathy   50

CHAPTER FIVE
Full Initiation of the Disease Reversal Process   **53**

Initial Protocol   53
Initial Quick Start Program   58
Plant Fiber   68
Raw Food is Nature's Way to Better Health   73

CHAPTER SIX
Complete Case Histories for Guidance through the Healing Process **79**

CASE HISTORY: Type 'A' Crohn's Disease (2006)   80
First Appointment   81
Patient's Daily Regime   85
Summary of Case History: Type 'A' Crohn's Disease Patient   94
A Common Diet Diet-Related Colitis Case History   98
Patient Testimonial   98
CASE HISTORY: Crohn's Disease/Fistula (2015) Following the Quick Start Program 100

CHAPTER SEVEN
**Replace Popular Medications with Safe and Effective
Natural Alternatives**   **109**

Natural Alternatives to Popular Pain Medication   109
Natural Alternatives for Antibiotics and Destroying Superbugs   113
Can Antibiotics Cause Crohn's Disease and Colitis?   114
Worldwide Concern of Antibiotic Overuse (WHO Agency Report)   114
How Do Patients Protect Themselves From Harmful and Deadly Germs? 115
Antibiotic Replacements That Are Safe and Effective   115

CHAPTER EIGHT
**Treating Depression and Stress Safely and Effectively
with Non-Drug Remedies**   **121**

The Stress Syndrome and Its Effects on Gut Diseases and the Body 121
Drug Free Ways to Aid Depression and Anxiety   127

Non-Drug Alternatives to Treat Depression   131
Discover Passionflower's Calming and Healing Benefits   133
Evidence for Medicinal Indications   134

CHAPTER NINE
Best Immune and Healing Support   137

What is Colostrum?   137
Probiotics Benefits Crohn's Disease and All Other Gastrointestinal Complaints   139
Monitoring Candida Benefits All Gut Disorders   141
Carrot Juice Quickens the Healing Process of Crohn's Disease
and All Other Gut Abnormalities   143
Other Common Deficiencies Related to Gut Dysbiosis   144
Aloe Vera Promotes Healing of Crohn's Disease
and Other Gastrointestinal Complaints   145

CHAPTER TEN
Necessary Elements for a Disease Reversal Process   147

Omega 3 Fatty Acids (EFAs) are Essential for Rebuilding Tissue
and Improving Longevity   147
Vitamin D Benefits Crohn's Disease and Other Similar Complications   151
Supplementation Overview   155
A List of Common Deficiencies   157
Tissue Salts   160
What Vitamins and Minerals are Lost with Crohn's Disease,
Colitis, Celiac, IBS and Chronic Diarrhea?   162

CHAPTER ELEVEN
Natural Remedies and Formulas for Healing Intestinal Tract Tissue 167

Herbal Recommendations   167
How to Make an Infusion or Decoction   168
The Benefits of Herbal Remedies   169
Additional Herbal Recommendations and Sample Formulas   172
Determining Dosage for Children   181
Herbal and Supplement Product Sources and Locations   183

CHAPTER TWELVE

Specific Dietary Protocols for Gastrointestinal Diseases 187

Acid and Alkaline Forming Foods for Typical Intestinal Disorders 187

Dietary Suggestions for Crohn's Disease, Ulcerative Colitis, and Celiac Disease 190

Suggested Foods 197

Treatment Plan for Colitis (Microscopic, Collagenous, and Lymphocytic Colitis) 209

Treatment Plan and Diet for Irritable Bowel Syndrome (IBS) 212

Daily Suggestions for IBS 215

Constipation Recommendations and Solutions 217

CHAPTER THIRTEEN

Best Choices for Gluten-Free Grains, Fiber and Foods 223

Gluten-Free Grains and Products 223

Additional Gluten-Free Flours and Thickeners 226

Gluten-Free Plant Fiber 227

Plants Related to Wheat that May be Tolerated by Celiac Patients 229

Other Related Items from Wheat Sources 230

Gluten-Free Flours 230

List of Gluten-Free Ingredients and Foods 232

CHAPTER FOURTEEN

Conclusion 235

Sample: Crohn's Disease and Gastrointestinal Complaint Questionnaire 238

About Hyperbaric Oxygen Treatment (HBOT) 239

Celiac Disease Critical Research Areas 241

Herbal Remedies: Additional Research Resources 243

Bibliography 245

About the Author 255

ACKNOWLEDGEMENTS

I wish to acknowledge all those who have supported me, and give a special thanks to everyone who played a part during the entire writing process. You will always be remembered in my heart.

I would like to acknowledge the skilled editoral team at Hatherleigh Press who worked their magic. I especially want to express my deep appreciation to Anna Krusinski, Ryan Kennedy, Andrew Flach and Ryan Tumambing. Thank you so much.

I am indebted to Dr. Ellen Tart-Jensen, who extended me a great honor by writing the foreword to this book, and who has always showed unwavering support to her students. You can read more about Ellen Tart-Jensen Ph.D. at www.bernardjensen.com.

A special note of thanks to my husband Ron for challenging me in the initial stages of writing, as well as for his encouragement and his assistance in helping this book reach fruition.

I applaud my case histories, who worked so diligently at turning their health around.

And to Jill, who also conquered her health challenges and wrote the testimonial of her experience, included in this book.

I am extremely appreciative to my test readers for their time and caring support: Doreen Valente, Joan Hutcheson, Pat Judd, Barbara Vos and Helen Gzik.

And to Doreen Valente, herself a nursing professor at St. Joseph Hospital School of Nursing, I thank you for your academic assistance and unwavering support throughout the whole of my career.

I appreciate my staff at Renew You, who supported and encouraged me throughout this publication, especially Lydia Waldropt and Rose Posteraro.

I would like to thank Karen McKnight for her guidance and continual support throughout the writing of this publication.

Lastly, I honor all authors whose expertise enables people to understand nutritional supplements, dietary change, and how to use the wonderful healing power of plants.

FOREWORD

IT IS WITH great pleasure that I write the foreword to this life changing book, *Reverse Gut Diseases Naturally*. The information in this book is extremely important, especially at this time in the history of both the United States and the world as a whole. Next to lung cancer, colon cancer is the second leading cause of death each year in the United States, as well as in Canada. In addition, millions more Americans and people world-wide suffer from some form of inflammatory bowel disease, including Crohn's disease, celiac, and diverticulitis. People are weary of needing to receive medication that only subdues or masks their symptoms without being provided with an understanding of the cause of their digestive disorders and a plan for healing that root cause.

The author, Michelle Honda, was inspired to study natural healing and nutrition due to her own personal health concerns. For years, Michelle suffered with chronic constipation, which eventually caused foul breath and skin eruptions. She tried antibiotics, to no avail, but found that when she began to include good portions of high fiber cereals into her diet, her constipation abated and normal bowel movements were achieved. The foul breath and skin eruptions disappeared. She also found that when she eliminated estrogen and started juicing and drinking raw vegetable juices, her health improved even further.

I met Michelle Honda many years ago, when she was one of my students studying nutrition, colon health, and iridology with me through Westbrook University and Bernard Jensen International. She was one of the brightest, most ambitious students I have ever had the privilege of teaching. I could tell she truly cared about her work and would go far in life working to eliminate pain and illness in others. Her coursework included the research of my father-in-law, the late Dr. Bernard Jensen, who wrote extensively on colon health in his books, *Tissue Cleansing Through Bowel Management* and *Better Bowel Care*. For sixty years, he was a pioneer in teaching good nutrition and colon cleansing throughout the United States, Canada, and over fifty different countries world-wide. During that time, I had the opportunity to work with him for several years at his "Hidden Valley Health Ranch," and saw people with some of the worst health conditions imaginable come back to vibrant health through juicing, eating organic foods, drinking pure water, and cleansing the colon. He always stated, "Nature will heal when given the opportunity." He was so successful in his work that he was awarded the Pax Mundi Award for World Peace and was knighted three times by the Knights of Malta.

Dr. Bernard Jensen studied the work of Sir Arbuthnot Lane, who is quoted within this book by Dr. Honda. Dr. Lane was a great English surgeon and physician to the English Crown. He specialized in bowel problems, and found when he surgically removed a section of the colon, not only did colon disease improve, but another illness that seemingly had no connection to the colon would go away. For example, when he removed a section of the colon in a boy who had been in a wheelchair for many years with arthritis, the boy completely recovered and was able to walk again six months after the operation. Another woman with goiter had a definite remission six months after a section of her bowels was removed. After many great results such as these, Dr. Lane began to see a relationship between the toxic bowel and the function of various organs in the body. He became very interested in changing and healing the bowels through dietary methods rather than surgery. He spent the next twenty-five years of his life teaching people how to take care of their intestinal tract through good nutrition, and not surgery. He came to believe that all maladies are due to the lack of good food principles, or else the absence of the normal defenses of the body, such as protective flora. He taught that when protective flora was absent, toxic bacteria invade the alimentary canal, creating poisons that then pollute the bloodstream. These poisons would then eventually deteriorate and destroy every tissue, gland, and organ of the body. And, as you will see reported throughout this book, this research still holds true today.

In my own natural healing and nutrition practice, I have seen the conclusions reached by Dr. Bernard Jensen and Sir Arbuthnot Lane proven again and again. When coaching mothers on how to help their children with chronic constipation, the mothers will report that, after the constipation goes away, other health problems such as ear infections, sinus congestion, frequent colds, and allergies clear up. Other times, when I have taught people with chronic constipation proper nutrition and how to cleanse and heal their colons, their psoriasis or arthritis will then disappear. Indeed, with good nutrition and colon cleansing, lower back pain, muscle aches, sore throats, headaches, and many other maladies have been shown to reliably improve.

Contained within these pages is one of the most thorough books on healing the intestinal tract through natural methods that I have ever seen. Dr. Bernard Jensen and Sir Arbuthnot Lane would be very proud of Dr. Michelle Honda, which is to say nothing of the pride I feel towards my former student. In addition to her formal studies from textbooks, Dr. Honda has been in the trenches with people suffering from health problems for many years. She has had tremendous experience with treating all kinds of conditions with proper nutritional protocols. Dr. Honda has specialized in problems of the intestinal tract, because she too has recognized that when the colon is healed, the whole body improves.

This book focuses on practically every bowel-related disease or problem one can have. She begins with a look at bowel inflammation, before delving into a thorough explanation of how the digestive process works. Dr. Honda reviews constipation, diarrhea, irritable bowel syndrome, leaky gut syndrome, abscesses, fistulas, colitis, Crohn's disease, celiac disease, candida, ulcerative colitis, diverticulitis, and much more. She discusses the depression and pain that are linked to bowel problems. Best of all, she provides information regarding the means of testing, specific foods, herbal remedies, juices, and lifestyle programs available for teaching one how to truly heal and live a healthy life. Whether you are a doctor, nurse, natural health care practitioner, nutritionist, chiropractor, or parent, this book will be beneficial to all. It is well written and thoroughly organized—a priceless treasure for these times.

—Ellen Tart-Jensen, Ph.D., D.Sc., C.C.I.I.
Author of *Health is Your Birthright:*
How to Create the Health You Deserve

PREFACE

A QUESTION THAT I have often been asked is, "Why are you writing a book on this subject?" For the average healthy person, there are far more so-called "in" topics to choose from, illnesses that are consistently in the forefront of the news media. But from a personal and professional perspective, I am all too aware of the many health issues which serve as inhibiting factors in regards to gastrointestinal diseases, all of which influence a person's healing process. As a practicing holistic doctor and author, there is a great need for a comprehensive book which also addresses the underlying concepts of these illnesses, and how to gain momentum in the healing process.

I want to teach my readers as I have taught my patients, explaining how the condition manifests and how the body works. Being proactive and taking part in the healing process is part of the learning process, the first step of which is realizing that their health problem is not restricted to the symptoms of their disease.

For this reason, the contents of this book include the main areas of imbalances, as well as common testing problems. For example, the body cannot produce sufficient energy when key organs and glands, such as the adrenals and thyroid, are functioning at far less than optimum levels. These glands, along with their amino acids and hormones, affect our mood-enhancing brain chemicals, coping skills, metabolism, circulation and energy output.

Traditional medicine does not offer information on how to nutritionally support the body or these glands. Being that thyroid testing is less than adequate, I have expanded on the latest testing methods to help you understand this process and better protect yourself against misinformation.

It cannot be ignored that one of the main inhibitors to good health is the patient themselves. Even after learning how best to protect their health, people still cling to their old ways and habits. The hope is that at some point, many of these individuals will wake up to the fact that it is up to them to take action and apply these lifestyle changes and treatment therapies, which are designed to return them to a time when they were happy with their life and health.

Early on in my practice, I recognized the need for information that would prevent the onset of health problems, as well as viable solutions to put people back into the driver's seat of their own health. I began writing for local papers, magazines and other publications. For several years I was prompted by patients, staff and those who were aware of my work to write a book on how to treat the chronic conditions of gut diseases. Having dedicated my life to continued education and the sharing of knowledge to promote good health, my goal is to truly help people on their journey to better health, regardless of their health challenge. Whether patients are suffering with diabetes, heart disease, cancer, ADHD, autism, or gut dysbiosis as found in this book, my intention is to introduce them to safe options when dealing with health issues, and to help them live longer and happier lives.

I encourage all of my patients and friends to pass along what they have learned about supporting the body and its balance. In addition, I seek to share the alternative of complementary medicine and therapies for all the many commonly prescribed medications. For example, for those who suffer from depression, anxiety, pain and inflammation, there are several natural, effective solutions that do not produce side effects. And all of this is besides the escalated need for viral and superbug remedies that are both safe and effective. The need for such information is widespread, and is in fact reaching a critical point in modern society.

The general public cannot fathom the health care costs for the treatment of digestive system disorders. Besides the question of fiscal expense, the day to day difficulty of managing a busy lifestyle, all the while feeling hampered in every direction you turn, takes its own toll. If you have ever been involved in the life of someone who is actually coping with a debilitating condition, you will understand why all they want is to be normal.

The information in this publication embraces the whole body and all aspects of gut dysbiosis. A diet plan could help to suppress many of the gut-wrenching symptoms caused by gut disease, but if the person is still suffering with chronic depression, for example, they cannot be said to be fully healed. There must be balance in all areas of the person's life. With balance comes the ability to direct and steer one's own path; the opportunity not to be a bystander, watching life pass them by.

Our research and health sciences are consistently making incredible strides and advances in the areas of cell biology and environmental sciences, including phytochemistry. Of particular interest to me, at least, are the new discoveries being made regarding special properties in plants that offer tremendous nutritional and medicinal value. And yet I virtually never see any of these wonderful discoveries in the news media or in the weekly papers.

As a society, we have gone from having muscle aches and pains, brought on by a hard day's work, to having multiple diseases at far younger ages, in what *should* be the prime of our life. It isn't uncommon for me to see a patient that has several diseases or health complaints.

I learned at a young age that the state of our nutrition affects how we feel. I was exposed to completely life-changing diseases in family members. I have also learned just how little people know about what their body requires, on a nutritional level, to maintain peak performance. It wasn't hard to see the effects of certain medications and a lifetime of bad habits, coupled with inadequate nutrition. These outcomes are sadly very predictable.

When explaining a patient's condition, and the way it manifested through stages of disruption and imbalance, the same scenarios repeat themselves. The patient is informed about the real need for their involvement in the healing process, making them aware of what it will take to fully reverse their condition and return them to health. The more compromised one's health situation, the more attention is required in all areas of body weaknesses and lifestyle, including diet and any habits that could otherwise sabotage your success.

So, what is needed to help avoid these scenarios continuing to repeat themselves? First and foremost, education, preferably during our academic years, is needed to provide us with a good baseline on how to feed our bodies, so our body's systems can rebuild, repair and function optimally. Hopefully in time this much needed knowledge will be brought to the forefront of our medical institutions and educational systems. Until then, awareness and quality information is accessible only through the work of publishers that have dedicated their livelihoods to providing information enabling alternate lifestyle choices and alternative treatment solutions to assist people in reclaiming their health. Authors and practitioners owe an immense debt of gratitude to publishers like Hatherleigh Press for their commitment to a better environment, healthier food choices and the freedom to choose your health care modality, so that future generations may benefit from their efforts.

Throughout this book, you will find solutions and guidance regarding all the stages and related illnesses that typically develop around gut inflammation. My goal for this book is to help guide and support you through all the problems that a patient will typically encounter in the healing process and maintenance of gut disorders.

Among the tools and topics covered in this book are:

1. Understanding the disease process through all of its stages.

2. Various diseases and conditions, including Crohn's disease, ulcerative colitis, collagenous colitis, celiac, irritable bowel syndrome, diverticulitis, chronic diarrhea, leaky gut, constipation, fistulas and abscesses.

3. Initial protocols, including a quick start program to quickly address the worst symptoms.

4. How to start and continue the reversal process.

5. Methods for empowering the body to heal, including:

    • Correcting nutritional deficiencies
    • Finding the most effective supplements that heal and nourish the body
    • Non-drug solutions for pain, inflammation, depression, anxiety, diarrhea, bleeding, gas, bloating, spasms, nausea and more
    • Diet protocol for each condition
    • Removing one or several triggers for over-reactive immune response
    • Treatment for emotional, anxiety and stress issues
    • Dietary and supplementation that promote speedier healing and recovery
    • Natural killers of viruses and bacteria, fungus and yeast
    • Strong immune boosters
    • Blood purifying and detoxification
    • The best herbal healing formulas
    • Up to date lists of gluten-free flours, ingredients and foods

6. An extreme Type "A" Crohn's patient case history (with severe complications), including step-by-step details of the patient's healing process, as well as a case history involving Crohn's disease and a fistula that fully healed in five weeks following the Quick Start Program.

One need only look at the alarming statistics throughout North America and other industrialized countries to understand the great necessity for prevention and for treatment that will actually alleviate and reverse the symptoms associated with most gut disorders. Current reports show an estimated 1 percent (or 1 in 133) of Americans endure celiac disease. Approximately ten years ago, it was estimated that IBD (inflammatory bowel disease) had touched approximately 50 million Americans. As of 2004, ulcerative colitis had affected as many as 400,000 Americans, with most cases of ulcerative colitis developing in patients between the ages of 15 and 35 (although children and older adults also develop the disease). Crohn's disease is also on the rise in the United States, distressing 150 out of 100,000 persons.

The statistics and health care costs of digestive system disorders pretty much speak for themselves in regards to the need for more helpful information. These statistics, along with the percentage of patients I see with digestive complaints, is the main reason why I have chosen to write on this topic, over the myriad other disorders that are life threatening and life changing.

I hope this book brings you encouragement and guidance on the path to reclaiming your health.

—Michelle Honda, PhD.D.Sc.

CHAPTER ONE

Common Denominators for Chronic Digestive Complaints

Bowel Disorders are Related to Other Disease Complaints

The evidence that we have today supports what Dr. Bernard Jensen noticed many years ago: that bowel complaints have a direct effect upon other specific organs in the body. Dr. Sir Arbuthnot Lane, a surgeon for the King of England whose specialty was bowel problems, noticed the same thing. He became extremely proficient at removing sections of the bowels, a procedure which gained him a worldwide reputation. While continuing this work, he began to notice a peculiar occurrence: he observed patients recovering from other diseases that had no apparent connection to the colonic surgery. For example, a young boy who suffered from arthritis for many years, and who was in a wheelchair at the time of surgery, recovered entirely from the arthritis only six months after the procedure. Another case history involved a woman with a goiter: again, when Dr. Lane removed a specific section of the bowel in surgery, there followed a definite remission of the goiter within six months. It became evident to him that there was a connection between toxic bowels and the functioning of various organs in the body.

These findings intrigued him so much that he became interested in changing the bowels through dietary means. Consequently, he spent the remainder of his career and life teaching people how to properly care for their bowels through nutrition, and not just by surgery. Sir Lane states, "All maladies are due to the lack of certain food principles, such as mineral salts or vitamins, or the absence of the normal defenses of the body, such as the natural protective flora. When this occurs, toxic bacteria invade the lower alimentary canal, and the poisons thus generated pollute the bloodstream and gradually deteriorate and destroy every tissue, gland and organ of the body."

Dr. John Harvey Kellogg (1855–1946), known for being unconventional and innovative for his time, embraced vegetarianism and wrote a book on hydrotherapy. As Dr. Kellogg extended his expertise into colon care and hygiene, he began practicing a diet of whole grains, yogurt, fruits, salads and cheeses. He also brought awareness of friendly bacteria within the bowels, which aid the colon in reducing putrefaction and fermentation. Dr. Kellogg determined that the bowels should be approximately 85 percent *acidophilus bacteria* and 15 percent *bacillus coli*. This is an accurate bacterial balance for a healthy bowel. Regrettably, this ratio is about opposite for most people living in North America. (The exception to this rule would be of those individuals who traditionally eat kefir, yogurt or take a prepared probiotic supplement purchased from a health food store.)

Assessing the Problems of Intestinal Health

Debilitating and distressing intestinal complications have plagued mankind for years. The labeling of these conditions may have changed over the years, along with the methods of diagnosis, care and treatment. However, one common factor has remained strong throughout the centuries—diet plays a significant role, not only in treating and curing these conditions, but also in determining their origins. Disorders such as Crohn's disease, colitis, celiac, irritable bowel syndrome, diverticulitis, constipation, chronic diarrhea, and cancer are all directly affected by the substances taken into the body.

A quick glimpse into the prevalence of Inflammatory Bowel Disease (IBD) in North America shows the United States on a fast track for IBD, with a reported 1.4 million Americans having been diagnosed with Crohn's or colitis, most before the age of 30. These conditions are represented by inflammation (redness and swelling) and ulceration (sores) of the small and large intestines. Just as distressing, reports confirm that celiac disease and irritable bowel syndrome (IBS) are globally on the rise. (For updates, contact the Information Resource Center at 888-694-8872.)

The need for a permanent solution and greater awareness is undeniable, particularly in view of the steadily increasing statistics for all gastrointestinal disorders. Popping pills in response to symptoms, all while having your questions regarding dietary causes dismissed by your phyisciain, will not assist you in ultimately conquering these aliments.

As a format for treating your gut complaints, this book addresses the primary functioning of your immune system, working to strengthen it while calming its auto-immune response. Additionally, certain glands which play a paramount role in your disease reversal and future health, and which are instrumental for supplying energy and mood enhancement, will be targeted for improvement. When your body is weak and malnourished, it does not have the strength and capacity to bring about your ultimate goal of symptom-free health.

The Healing Power of Plants

Over the last several decades, intense effort has been made to discover new and innovative therapeutic organic compounds which are effective against otherwise medication-resistant germs. Medicinal plants have been increasingly incorporated into cosmetics, food supplements and pharmaceuticals. But, as medications cannot grow tissue, our bodies cannot be expected to fully heal without help from our diet, along with some extra supplementation to correct major imbalances. And, since medications are the most familiar form of treatment to Americans, an alternative must be provided to expedite the healing process, one that is safe and free of side effects.

Often times, mild to severe symptoms of anxiety, depression, pain and inflammation accompany more problematic gut dysbiosis complaints, all of which are fully remedied within this book. Also included are the best remedies available for replacing antibiotics.

Leaky Gut Triggers Auto-Immune Response

For example, one of the physical attributes of Crohn's disease and other gut complaints is leaky gut syndrome and permeable tissue lining. As a result of these holes in the gut, unwanted particles pass through the lining of the stomach into the blood. Substances such as gluten protein, once in the blood, serve as a signal to the immune system to attack and destroy. If this occurrence is continually repeated, the offending protein eventually becomes recognized as an immune response trigger, and becomes classified by the immune system as a foreign and harmful element. This is an example of a process that can precipitate an allergic reaction, even though the person was not originally inherently predisposed. The gut lining must be healed over to prevent leakage of foreign material that could otherwise initiate this immune response.

This is initially a two step process: first, the substances which trigger the immune response must be removed until such time as the body has healed and no longer recognizes the substance as harmful. During this elimination process, the gut can begin the reversal process of promoting tissue integrity once again. This is the second step, accomplished by supporting the immune system and the body with healing and health promoting substances. The information and therapies needed to support an accelerated healing process are discussed in Chapter 11. Further details are provided in Chapter 12 for reintroducing the original trigger substances.

The Diet's Crucial Influence

While the classification of gut-related complaints has almost certainly changed over time, so too have the lifestyle factors which influence them, along with the unfortunate addition of certain dietary assaults and harmful agents like drugs and the exposure to environmental toxins. All of the nutrients used by our body (with the exception of oxygen and water) are absorbed through our food intake.

Many acute and chronic health disorders have been traced back to, or are in some way associated with, gut dysbiosis. A number of health professionals feel that many diseases may originate in the gut and bowel area. For example, more than forty percent of Crohn's disease patients have subsequently developed lactose intolerance. Disorders such as Crohn's disease, colitis, celiac, irritable bowel syndrome, diverticulitis, constipation, chronic diarrhea, gastritis and cancer are greatly influenced by our diet. Colon cancer, as an example, has been shown to have a direct correlation to constipation, and holds the second highest death rate of all cancers in Canada.

Research has revealed that a diet high in refined carbohydrates and low in fiber prolongs the transit time of bowel waste, resulting in greater production of putrefactive bacteria in the bowels. This information supports conditions including constipation, diverticulitis and even cancer; however, as a component, food is of far greater significance for those who suffer from Crohn's, colitis, celiac, irritable bowel syndrome and diarrhea.

With diet, and the resulting need for healthy habits in one's day-to-day life, it has become all the more important that patients with intestinal disorders receive the information and advice they need from medical professionals. And yet, time and again patients have come to me, saying that they were told there was no cause of or cure for their ailment. Ignorance is no longer an excuse in this area of medicine; the general public is learning and seeking not only answers and solutions, but practitioners who can assist them in healing their complaints. All areas of a person's life, including their family and friends, are affected by severe gut dysbiosis conditions. As such, normalcy is the number one goal of virtually every patient I see. They require not only advice and medical treatment, but counseling as well, which can oftentimes be helpful in bringing about understanding, while lessening the anxiety associated with the symptoms of bowel disorders.

I have great empathy for the thousands who suffer from these debilitating ailments, many of whom are still desperately in search of solutions, as well as an explanation as to why their bodies are reacting the way they are. Since bowel related problems are often very personal in nature and do not make for pleasant conversation, most people remain in the dark about this subject. As a result, our elimination process is one of the most important and often times neglected system in our bodies.

Symptoms are often intermittent and unpredictable, with no singular cure or treatment. Nevertheless, evidence is mounting from testimonials and test results showing vast improvement in a patient's condition relating to how, when and what we eat, which trigger reactions that are unique to each individual. As to the level of severity, it depends on various other factors, such as inherent weaknesses, allergies, sensitivities, emotional and physical stress levels, state of health and attitude, all of which play an important part.

The Origin of Crohn's and Colitis Complaints

A brief look into the origins of the symptoms of Crohn's disease and ulcerative colitis shows that those people suffering with chronic gut disorders are not necessarily born with an inherent weakness—a few of my patients have had Crohn's develop purely from emotional stress. However, the far more common culprits are the problems resulting from antibiotics and food intolerances.

The following is a series of events within a gut diagnosed with Crohn's and severe complications of colitis:

- Food intolerance results in the inability to digest sugars from carbohydrates.
- Incapacity to digest sugars and absorption of disaccharides results in malabsorption.
- Bacterial overgrowth produces by-products that injure intestinal walls.
- Excessive mucus production from irritating microbial overgrowth impairs digestion.
- Imbalance of gut micro flora. The gut becomes overrun with yeast and damaging micro-organisms, promoting degeneration of intestinal walls.

One main focus of dietary programs is determining the offending substances which are denying the microbial bacteria the nourishment they need to proliferate within the intestines. Malnourishment is common among people suffering with inflammatory bowel disease (IBD). By using (primarily) pre-digested carbohydrates, a person with intestinal problems can have maximum nourishment without contributing to the intestinal microbe population. Supplementation and easily digested foods and liquids are necessary to combat nutrient loss through diarrhea, pain and nausea.

While colon stagnation is traditionally induced by constipation, the opposite holds true in conditions such as inflammatory bowel disorders, irritable bowel syndrome, celiac, and diarrhea. In order for the body to properly absorb and make use of the food you put in it, it requires adequate time in between assimilation, and evacuation of those nutrients. However, in situations where the body reacts violently to eliminate an offending substance, the body loses out on otherwise available nutrients. Persistent gas, bloating and diarrhea are common companions to this occurrence. Another culprit triggering inflammation in the gastrointestinal tract is fungi, through their production of mycotoxins. Mycotoxins have been linked to the development of leaky gut syndrome and have shown to initiate many autoimmune diseases.

The purpose of this publication is to highlight the many benefits of natural healing methods and substances, without the problematic side effects of drugs. We need to adopt a lifestyle of *educating*, not medicating, as the saying goes. Many patients are not receiving adequate care as a direct result of lack of knowledge, both on their part, and on the part of the professionals treating and advising them on their condition. Typically health professionals treat the symptoms of intestinal disorders with drug related treatments rather than nutritionally based therapies. All too often, surgery becomes necessary, which in most cases can only provide temporary relief, and will usually necessitate a permanent lifestyle change (such as with a colostomy).

Medications Increase Nutritional Requirements

Despite being designed as a remedy, prescription medications have their own list of complications. The most common drugs used in the allopathic treatment of bowel disorders are corticosteroids and sulphasalazines. Both of these medications are known to increase the nutritional requirements of the body. For example, corticosteroids are known to stimulate the decomposition of proteins (catabolism), hinder protein formation and decrease the absorption of calcium and phosphorus, while increasing the urinary excretion of vitamin C, calcium, potassium, and zinc. In addition, they increase blood glucose levels, serum triglycerides and serum cholesterol, and increase the requirements for vitamin B6, ascorbic acid, folate and vitamin D. Corticosteroids have also shown to decrease bone formation and impede wound healing. Sulphasalazine medications have revealed restrictions in the assimilation and transport of folate, or folic acid, a B vitamin commonly found in liver and vegetables. Sufla drugs also reduce serum folate and iron, while escalating the urinary excretion of ascorbic acid. Throughout this book, we'll be giving special attention to the recommended supplementation needed to replace the nutrients lost through diarrhea and malabsorption.

Investigating the Causes and Triggers of Gut Complaints
Finding the origin and trigger of gut complaints involves investigation on the part of the practitioner, as well as full involvement on the part of the patient when initiating the reversal process, and in ultimately establishing complete recovery from these conditions. More awareness and education is needed, both among physicians and the general public. We cannot mask these diseases; we must do our due diligence and adapt around our intolerances. For many of those desiring to achieve and sustain normality, know that it *is* attainable through the proper management of diet and lifestyle.

Others will require additional help from complementary medicine and supplementation, especially in the initial stages. The digestive system is unique to each individual, and needs to be treated as such.

Longterm illness or more severe conditions (as seen with inflammatory bowel diseases) puts a greater responsibility on the patient, while incorporating appropriate time allowance for the healing process. The same may be said of the healing process as described by Hering's Law of Cure: "All cure starts from the inside out, and in the reverse order as the symptoms appeared." Understanding the basics of bowel anatomy and physiology will give us further insight into the causes and effects of the many substances that routinely are taken into our bodies and absorbed.

CHAPTER TWO

Empowering the Body to Heal

The Goal of the Digestive Process

The average person could not begin to describe how food is broken down and utilized within the body. The ways in which food is transformed by our body's enzymes into digestible matter, their individual roles in the body…these things just don't occur to most people. And yet, during a normal lifetime as much as sixty thousand pounds of food will pass through your digestive system. It is the purpose of our digestive system to extract essential nutrients from the food we consume, including proteins, quality fats, carbohydrates, vitamins, minerals and water. Our body's cells need these nutrients in order to reproduce and sustain our body at its optimum state of health and performance.

Digestion ultimately starts with the brain. The only conscious function we perform in digestion is chewing and swallowing. Normally, it should take food 18 hours after entering the stomach to continue on through to its completion stage, where it is ready for elimination. The normal rhythm of our body's muscular contraction (known as peristalsis) moves food along the entire digestive system, beginning with the esophagus. Upon reaching the stomach, digestive acids kick into action and begin breaking down the food particles into a consistency called chyme. Once food forms a chyme consistency, it then enters the first part of the small intestine (called the duodenum). The term "small intestine" is a bit of a misnomer; the name is derived from its narrow diameter, as the intestinal tract itself is approximately 21 feet in length, extending from the stomach to the large intestine.

Once in the duodenum, chyme is broken down by enzymes excreted by the pancreas, along with bile from the gallbladder. It is in this part

9

of the small intestine (the duodenum and jejunum) that the majority of absorption takes place. The contents continue on through to the ileum (the final section of the small intestine) for further nutrient extraction, with the assistance of many finger-like extensions called villi, which cover the surface of the small intestine. Chyme is then broken down into amino acids, simple sugars and fatty acids. These newly formed components are now ready for absorption via the bloodstream. The blood continues its journey to the liver for additional changes and utilization, where it is prepared for distribution to cells throughout the body.

Approximately 8–10 hours after eating, the food we eat will have advanced through the small intestine, and is mainly digested. The hard-to-digest parts of our meal now enter the large intestine and the colon, where the remaining indigestible matter will pass along the colon as feces. The colon is divided into segments: the cecum, ascending, transverse, descending, sigmoid and the rectum. The large colon is approximately five feet in length and two and a half inches in diameter. Unlike the small intestine, the large colon has a smooth mucous lining with a muscular layer encircling the mucosal inside layer. These muscles are called haustras, and it is their job to contract, allowing for considerable expansion. The peristaltic action propels the fecal matter toward the rectum and anus for elimination from the body.

Recommended Diet for Healthy Digestion

For proper colonic muscular activity to take place, the body must have adequate quantities of complex carbohydrates, (fruits, vegetables, legumes and grains). Note that fiber is not a food type in and of itself; rather, it is a variety of plant material, some of which *does* resist digestion. Incorporating more plant fibers into your diet will result in an increase in fecal mass, which in turn will require less transit time through the body, while providing material for the bowel muscle to knead upon. In other words, it gives your body more raw material to work with when eliminating waste from your body. Refined carbohydrates, by contrast, form soft, fiberless stools, which are more difficult for the bowel to propel along. In addition, white flour products have often been referred to as "wallpaper paste" within the gut; the sticky mass hinders the peristaltic action of our digestive tract, causing the waste inside to stagnate. The longer the transit time, the less water is absorbed, causing compacted fecal matter resembling hard, small stools. (Refer to Chapters 5 and 13 for information on plant fiber and gluten-free fiber.)

By adding complex carbohydrates to one's daily eating regime, one will experience an increase in energy levels, reduced blood cholesterol levels and more stable blood glucose measurements. Our current medical literature is full of reports supporting the beneficial effects of diet change in conjunction with intestinal disorders, heart disease, diabetes and cancer. Nor is this breaking news—a pioneering 12th century physician, Maimonides stated, "Man should always strive to have his intestines relaxed all the days of his life."

Thyroid and Adrenal Gland Support

The endocrine system is one of our body's most crucial systems. It consists of nine separate glands, which together secrete dozens of hormones into our bloodstream to regulate and support all the systems in the body. In this chapter, we'll be focusing primarily on the thyroid gland, below the larynx (voice box), with lobes lying on either side of the trachea, and the adrenal glands, which lie on top of the kidneys. Even though the body is to be (and indeed *should* be) treated as a whole, these two glands have a great effect on how we feel and cope when it comes to energy levels, cravings, stress, mood swings, patience, anger and anxiety. The endocrine system works as a team (although the thyroid, adrenals and pancreas actually work as a triad). For this reason, I have included information on how to support this area of the endocrine, as these glands—when either imbalanced or malnourished—have a huge impact on how we feel and how we manage our lives on a day-to-day basis (all of which impacts our healing process).

Thyroid Gland

As a natural medicine practitioner, I have long been aware that lab tests do not tell the whole story. The traditional thyroid test performed at the doctor's office serves as an example of a patient's signs and symptoms not correlating to the test results. The thyroid gland plays a significant role throughout the body, with every cell in the body having a thyroid hormone receptor. As it happens, the number one imbalance I see, and which most people are unaware of as being a concern or having an impact on their health, is hypothyroidism (underactive thyroid function). None of which is helped by patients being consistently told that their thyroid is working well!

How Does the Thyroid Gland Affect My Health?

Often referred to as the most abused gland in the body, the thyroid has earned this reputation because it is viewed as an emotional gland. Any episodes of great stress, sadness, anger, grief, lifestyle change or other stimulus can seriously burden this gland, creating an enormous nutritional need in order to keep up with the body's demand. Hypothyroidism can be looked at as a silent epidemic; however, hyperthyroidism is quickly climbing the list as an equal partner in many disturbances throughout the body. Listed below are some of the responsibilities of the thyroid gland:

1. Regulator: affects all parts of the body from the neck down and is responsible for the entire body's metabolism
2. Circulation: common symptoms of cold hands and feet, onto the more serious condition of Raynaud's Disease
3. Sexual: low libido, hormone production, energy, menstrual complaints, infertility, sexual dysfunction
4. Energy: low energy, fatigue, poor attitude
5. Weight gain: resting metabolic rate will be low, causing weight gain.
6. Required for athletic performance and a necessary component for achieving lean muscle mass, as seen with body builders
7. Immune function: over or under-reactive, allergies, autoimmune diseases
8. Removal of waste products
9. Reduced production of all hormones
10. Hair loss and the more severe form of alopecia
11. Skin: circles under the eyes, dry, acne, darker spots
12. Brain: mental sluggishness, poor memory, insomnia, depression, lack of focus, poor concentration
13. Vascular: high and low blood pressure, circulation
14. Fluid retention

The TSH Test: How Accurate Is It?

The Thyroid Stimulating Hormone Test (TSH) is a routine blood test done to check how well your thyroid gland is functioning. Unfortunately, tests are not always conclusive, and the TSH is a prime example of an inaccurate test. Many doctors have given reasons why this particular test is insufficient in producing an accurate reading.

The following are a few reasons, listed by Dr. J. Krop in his book *Healing the Planet One Patient at a Time*, as to why there are quite often negative blood results but positive clinical symptoms, when performing a thyroid TSH test.

- The blood sample represents a hormone level only at the moment it was taken. A 24 hour urine collection and analysis of hormones may give a more reliable result.

- T3 and free T4 blood tests sometime give an idea of what is in the blood, but don't really measure the amount of hormone in the cells.

- Research volunteers, on the basis of whom norms are established, do not necessarily have normal levels.

- The range of normal values is wide, so any value should be compared to the median range of values.

- Decreased blood volume due to arterial vasoconstriction, slow lymphatic drainage, muscopolysaccharide infiltration of vessel walls could all result in inaccurate results.

- TSH levels will only be elevated when the hypothalamus and pituitary gland are not myxedematous, and thyroid hormone levels are very low as seen in advanced cases.

- Hormone disruptors can block the cell receptors.

- Finally, never trust any test to be 100 percent accurate.

—Reprinted by Permission of Dr. Josef Krop

Further Comments from Dr. Krop

On October 15, 2014, Dr. J. Krop and I had a conversation about the correlation between adrenal fatigue and its effect on thyroid function. In addition to inadequate testing, Dr. Krop stated that adrenal function must be established and corrected *first* before the thyroid gland can function properly. He continued to say that the hormones secreted by the adrenal glands play crucial roles throughout the body, some of which are directly related to thyroid health and gonads. Dr. Krop also indicated that determining the factors causing stress to the adrenal glands, many of which are internal imbalances such as gut inflammation and digestion problems and a weak immune system, is crucial. Other factors to consider include constant emotional stressors, such as the chronic threat of loss (of a job, financial security, or a loved one) and the persistent day-to-day occurrences that ultimately deplete our glands and body. Psychological stress is only part of the problem, which in and of itself will cause adrenal fatigue. Environmental stressors are another component, including air pollution, household molds, pathogens, radiation (EMFs), and toxins such as pesticides and fungicides.

Other Factors Related to Thyroid Disorders
The following is a list of circumstances and conditions that can impact TSH levels.

- Pain and inflammation
- Food intolerances (especially gluten) and/or thyroid food inhibitors
- Adrenal exhaustion and excess cortisol or low cortisol levels
- Nutrient deficiencies
- Low hydrochloric acid: affects red blood cells from adequately distributing thyroid hormone
- Stress
- CFS (Chronic Fatigue Syndrome)
- Depression, PTSD (post traumatic disorder), schizophrenia
- Insulin resistance and diabetes
- Fibromyalgia
- Obesity and dieting too often
- Leptin resistant: A hormone expressed in the hypothalamus; a regulator of food and body weight
- Aging process
- Anemia

Adrenal Stress Inhibits Conversion of T4 to T3

There are many reasons why adrenal stress reduces the conversion of T4 to T3 (the two hormones excreted by the thyroid which play a large role in metabolism), and why weak adrenals can cause hypothyroid symptoms, even when the thyroid does not show any deficiencies itself. One example involves adrenal stress disrupting the hypothalamic, pituitary and adrenal axis (HPA). Chronic stress has also been shown to depress hypothalamic and pituitary function. Realizing that these two organs direct thyroid function, any interruption of the HPA axis will also suppress thyroid function.

A Closer Look at Thyroid Testing

Implications surrounding the thyroid's health far surpass the normal doctor's office thyroid test. The test itself has fallen under intense scrutiny among medical professionals *and* the general public, looking to see why this "Gold Standard Test" is not accurately reflecting the physical symptoms described by the patients. Anyone approaching this subject may be surprised by the many thyroid-related conditions and related causes. And the information surrounding the test and the thyroid's role in our health only become more complex the further you go.

After reviewing comments made by Dr. Kent Holtof, the problems surrounding the thyroid test are seen to extend beyond the list provided by Dr. Krop. Generally, a patient requests help and diagnosis with symptoms such as fatigue, weight gain, hair loss, cold hands and feet, heavy menses, hot flashes and brain fog, and noticeable decreases in memory.

Upon follow-up blood test results for the thyroid gland, the patient is most often told they are fine. But in truth, they are *not* fine; the standard TSH test is actually looking at a hormone produced by the pituitary gland. TSH governs the thyroid gland on the amount of hormone needed by the body. Upon examining test results, high TSH levels indicate low amounts of thyroid hormone, while low TSH levels indicate too much hormone. The problem is that these values fall under "typical," a reference which is far from accurate.

Relationship Between FT4, FT3, RT3 and TSH

Free T4 (FT4), an inactive form of T4 largely viewed as a storage vessel, must first be converted to Free T3 (the active form) for the body to maintain energy levels, as well as to both enhance and sustain metabolism. When undergoing thyroid testing at the doctor's office, make sure to request that both free and total levels of T4 and T3 are obtained, and confirm that your doctor is analyzing the free levels. The reason for checking free levels of T4 is to determine the amount of Free T4 that is available for conversion to T3; otherwise, T4 remains bound to proteins in the blood.

Another aspect to consider regarding thyroid testing are the overall levels of Reverse T3 (RT3). This variety of hormone is the "inactive" form of T3, made from storage hormone T4 via the liver, and has anti-thyroid effects. An excess of RT3 has an inhibiting effect on T4, essentially blocking its absorption into the body's cells. The result is thyroid functionality at less than optimum levels. This may be due to physiological reasons, such as by the adrenal glands producing too much or too little cortisol, and ferritin (iron) levels, which induce the body to create excess RT3 hormone. High cortisol levels inhibit the conversion of T4 to T3. Vitamin B12 levels may also play a role. All the physical anomalies related to stressed adrenals that lower red blood cell count can be considered contributing factors to increased levels of RT3.

In 2005, the Journal of Clinical Endocrinology and Metabolism published a study titled "Reverse T3 is the best measurement of thyroid tissue levels." The article stated that, "...the T3/rT3 ratio is the most useful marker for tissue hypothyroidism and as a marker of diminished cellular functioning." It further added that, in the presence of illness or physiological disorders such as depression and stress or obesity, "...look to the ratio between Free T3 (FT3) and Reverse T3 (RT3)."

How to Naturally Lower RT3 Levels
When looking to lower one's RT3 levels without resorting to medication, start with a liver cleansing program. A thorough liver cleanse will also involve a gall bladder cleanse, and is typically accomplished through a day-long fast from food, followed by a combination of olive oil and lemon juice (there are also programs incorporating salt and olive oil). Search online, or else ask your doctor regarding liver and gall stone cleansing programs.

Herbs such as milk thistle and dandelion, when taken over time while monitoring your RT3 levels, can also be effective (although the normal recommended dosage may require doubling). In addition, low levels of selenium have shown to increase RT3 hormone. (In such cases, take 100 mg of selenium daily.) Address adrenal function and identify stressors, and correct any adrenal insufficiency or fatigue.

Pregnant Women
Thyroid disorders are one of the most prevalent complications among pregnant women. An endocrine problem such as this can impact the health and well-being of the fetus, as well as promoting infertility and miscarriages. Monitor the thyroid gland closely.

Avoid Iodine for Hyperthyroidism (Thyroiditis/Hashimoto's Disease)
Similar to other thyroid conditions, the standard thyroid test may not include T3 levels. Since conventional testing typically measures T4 and thyroid stimulating hormone (TSH), without examining T3 levels, ensure this area of testing has been upgraded and properly considered. Remember that, in the incidence of hyperthyroidism and thyroiditis, the thyroid gland is releasing too much thyroid hormone.

Another area of testing is in regards to foods or substances that may be triggering an autoimmune response. Causes may involve problems with the immune system, food intolerances like gluten, bouts of high fever and Grave's disease (an autoimmune disorder). These conditions (as well as others) can cause hyperthyroidism. Cultures like the Japanese, who consume high amounts of iodine more often than others, are at risk for contracting Hashimoto's disease, also known as thyroiditis and inflammation of the thyroid. Medications such as interferon-alpha, interleudin-2, lithium and amiodarone can also bring about thyroiditis as a result of certain side effects.

Avoid: Baldderwrack (*Fucus vesiculosus*) and Ashwagandha (*Withania somnifera*).

Gluten Impacts the Thyroid Gland

When it comes to hyperthyroidism, it's best to consider treatment "through the back door." The key is to determine exactly what is triggering the immune response, while supporting the immune system and picking up as many deficiencies as possible. To calm down the autoimmune response, include higher amounts of magnesium in your diet, and remove gluten where possible. Gluten happens to have an almost identical matrix to thyroid tissue, which in turn causes the immune system to attack the protein gluten as well as the thyroid gland. In such cases extracts from herbs such as bugleweed have proven to be extremely valuable for the treatment of hyperthyroidism.

Sources for bugleweed include HerbPharm (www.herbpharm.com) and Sangsters (www.sangsters.com).

How Do I Care for the Thyroid Gland?

The thyroid gland requires a small amount of iodine daily in order to make thyroid hormone. It follows, then, that you should avoid iodine when the thyroid gland has become over active or inflamed until this condition is rectified. During the 1950s, the incidence rate of goiters (an enlarged, overworked thyroid) was such a problem that salt became iodized to ward it off. However, salt is *not* the ideal method of getting iodine into your system, and our soil has far fewer nutrients than in years previous. In other words, a supplement is required to feed this gland. The good news is that iodine is an inexpensive product to buy, and there are several natural sources, such as sea plants like kelp, dulse and seaweed, as well as convenient liquid iodine drops. Other choices include potassium iodide or full thyroid support in a combination product. These should be taken daily, as directed by the product of choice.

Nutrition for Disorders of the Thyroid Gland

Whether your thyroid condition is hypo or hyper, avoid sugar and caffeine products. Often times, people with low thyroid conditions turn to these stimulants to compensate for their lack of energy. In general, eat less starchy foods, carbs, sugar and sugar products (unless it is deemed safe, as for a diabetic), and eat more non-starchy vegetables and greens.

As I will continue to stress throughout this book, increasing your intake of omega 3 fatty acids in the form of fish oil and seed oils (such as flax seed) will greatly benefit your body. Your glands require high quality protein and fat. Other good fat sources include nuts and nut butters, avocados, seeds (like flax and sesame), olive oil, ghee, coconut oil and milk products, full fat and aged cheese, yogurt, kefir and cottage cheese.

Underactive Thyroid: Hypothyroidism
A lack of key nutrients can promote a thyroid condition, especially a hypo state. Adding quality supplements or herbs to increase intake of mineral and vitamins can help ease various deficiencies. Use whole food supplements whenever possible, such as those found in nutritional yeasts—all B vitamins and amino acids; algae (blue or green works best as a complete food source); raw juices for antioxidants, nutrition and enzymes; and sea vegetables or algae for trace minerals and iodine. Vitamin D3, selenium, zinc, alpha lipoic acid and magnesium should also be considered.

L-Tyrosine and L-Glutamine

L-Tyrosine is an amino acid earmarked for the thyroid gland which, during times of under-activity, offers more than one benefit. Most often, amino acids are tied into the neurotransmitters of the brain. In the instance of L-Tyrosine, it is a required element for dopamine in the brain, a neurotransmitter responsible for any number of functions, including mood. Increasing the health of the thyroid, then, has a direct effect on one's mood; a win-win, all round. It is also responsible for the formation of two main adrenal hormones (epinephrine and adrenaline). L-Glutamine, another amino acid mentioned throughout this book, is required for cell replication of the intestinal tract. Similar to L-Tyrosine, L-Glutamine also interrelates a neurotransmitter, in this case glutamate. Glutamate interacts with L-Glutamine, promoting feelings of well-being among (several other functions.)

Note that L-Tyrosine is not recommended *during* hyper states or conditions of inflammation involving the thyroid gland, until these conditions have become balanced and rectified.

Thyroid Gland Sources: Most companies have combination products for glandular support. Suggestions for combination formulas are as follow: Natural Factors, Thorne, Now, Sangsters, Botanica, Eclectric Institute, Vitamin Shoppe Brand, Herb Pharm and several other companies. The United States also has several sources; including raw or desiccated thyroid and other glandular substances: Natural Sources, Solaray, Seroyal, NatraBio and others.

Thyroid Requires Probiotics for Function: Hypo or Hyper Thyroid State
Another essential dietary component for health maintenance and the functioning of the thyroid gland is the consumption of "probiotics" in sup-

plement form, or else in certain foods such as yogurt, kefir and clabbered milk. 20 percent of thyroid gland function depends on friendly flora.

For hyperthyroidism, avoid all refined foods, dairy products, wheat, gluten, sugar, caffeine, coffee, alcohol and other chemical stimulants.

For Hashimoto's Disease (Thyroiditis)
Glutathione is a potent antioxidant and has demonstrated great benefit as an immune modulator. It has shown to help regulate and strengthen the immune system while dampening autoimmune response with conditions like Hashimoto's disease. Among its many benefits, glutathione promotes healing and protection to thyroid tissue.

Adrenal Glands

The adrenal glands are small glands that lie on top of the kidneys. These very hard working glands have often been likened to overachievers, and are responsible for regulating our body's response to stress. As mentioned earler, regarding the thyroid, the thyroid, adrenals and pancreas work as a triad, always interrelated. Thus, even though the body is to be treated as a whole, the thyroid and adrenal glands and the hormones they produce greatly impact how we feel and cope when it comes to energy levels, cravings, stress, mood swings, water retention, weight gain and loss, patience, anger and anxiety. Adrenal dysfunction can also lead to food sensitivities, blood sugar imbalances and infections. Basically, the adrenal glands are involved in all perceived stressors that impact the body. A few examples of physiological effects due to the adrenal glands include hormonal balancing, gastrointestinal function, thyroid and immune function, bone metabolism and more.

Brain Connection
The adrenal glands consist of two main sections, described as the outer adrenal cortex and the inner adrenal medulla. The adrenal glands have a special connection to the brain (the medulla), as opposed to other glands, whose messages are related via hormone pathways. The medulla is a direct hotline of sorts, due to a nerve pathway connection from the brain to the inner medulla. The brain is so designed as to allow for rapid responses to stressful situations, such as when the flight-or-fight response is triggered.

Adrenal Gland Laboratory Testing

The adrenal salivary test is the most popular method for assessing adrenal function. It is simple enough: the patient takes four saliva samples throughout the course of their day. These samples help determine salivary cortisol and DHEA levels (although other factors need to be incorporated, like the patient's history and symptoms).

A study involving serum cortisol and salivary cortisol shows almost no difference in test results. A test conducted by ClinChem Lab in 1998 found that, "In 42 of the 45 tests performed, the same conclusion as to cortisol status was drawn when based on serum and salivary cortisol responses. In healthy subjects and good responders the mean cortisol relative increase was greater in saliva than in serum in all three tests."

Adrenal Gland Dysfunction

Overactive adrenal glands produce too much cortisol, epinephrine (adrenaline) and aldosterone, all of which may lead to insulin resistance and metabolic syndrome.

Underactive adrenal glands essentially do the opposite, producing inadequate amounts of hormones such as cortisol, which then interrupts the release of insulin, causing symptoms of hypoglycemia. Symptoms related to low blood sugar may be trembling, feeling light headed, impatience and irritability.

Symptoms of adrenal exhaustion are extreme fatigue and often accompanied by psychological stress. Adrenal fatigue is a collection of symptoms and indicators. For example, a person exhibiting extreme fatigue may crave salt and experience weakness in the legs. Prolonged and acute stress due to illnesses such as respiratory infections, influenza, bronchitis or pneumonia, can leave the adrenal glands depleted. Unfortunately, the symptom of fatigue is not relieved by sleep. Another scenario where adrenals become exhausted is in cases where the threat of death is looming, either by the person themselves or a care giver, such as a parent with a child dealing with a prolonged illness.

Neither is being overtired or weak the worst symptoms associated with adrenal fatigue. Feelings of being overwhelmed, coupled with the emotion of sadness and depression, add to an already weakened state. All too often, people suffering from adrenal fatigue or exhaustion routinely turn to stimulants like coffee and colas to get them through the day. Stress may also be compounded by and related to the frequent use of caffeine, alcohol, nicotine and medications. You may want to consider natural methods of propping up your adrenals if you regularly experience one or more of the following symptoms:

1. Fatigue or listlessness, in spite of adequate sleep

2. Still feeling tired in the morning, even when you've had eight hours of sleep

3. No "get up and go," feeling worn out and weighed down

4. Lacking the reserves to bounce back from stress or illness

5. Crave salt or sugar, eating binges

6. Lack of sleep as a result of insomnia

7. Sluggishness, especially in the morning and mid-afternoon (the thyroid gland reaches its low for the day at mid-afternoon)

8. Low libido or a decrease in sex drive

9. Requires a great deal of effort to do everyday tasks

10. Stress becomes overwhelming

11. Heightened PMS symptoms and increased weight gain

12. Brain fog, hard to focus or memory problems

13. Far less resistance to bacteria and virus invasion. Recovery time is much longer

14. Mild depression to feelings of desperation. Under these circumstances, a person will not experience much enjoyment or happiness in their life.

Can the Adrenal Glands Contribute To Weight Gain?

Other symptoms of low adrenals include higher than normal levels of cortisol (a stress hormone) which often signals fat storage. During this time, adrenaline may be over produced, creating more unwanted feelings. Overproduction of unwelcome substances like cortisol and other hormones needlessly overworks the glands, weakening them. This scenario may create sugar cravings and eating binges.

What Nutrients Assist the Adrenal Glands?

B5 (pantothenic acid) is earmarked for the adrenals. Full adrenal support and a B complex are also helpful. Glands in general want high quality protein and fats. Essential fatty acids (EFAs) are a type of good fat that the body requires for proper functioning and restoring. EFAs are always earmarked for the endocrine system as a whole, and each gland or organ individually.

In reference to "a full adrenal or full thyroid support," these are specialized combination products available through practitioners and some health food stores. This type of supplement offers more support. Products such as these may be a combination of desiccated glandular extracts or a combination of vitamins, minerals, herbs and amino acids. Most companies have combination products for glandular support and some even have raw or desiccated glandular extracts. The United States have several sources, including Natural Sources, Solaray, Seroyal, NatraBio and others. Combination formulas include Natural Factors, Thorne, Now, Sangsters, Eclectric Institute, Vitamin Shoppe Brand, Herb Pharm and several other companies.

Nutritional Recommendations for the Adrenal Glands

A broad range of vitamins and minerals should be considered when supporting the adrenal glands. Adequate nutrition through diet and supplements will lower cortisol output while aiding and relieving stress (while also reducing cravings). These include:

- Omega 3 fatty acids in adequate amounts (refer to Chapter 10: Omega 3 Fatty Acids (EFAs) are Essential for Rebuilding Tissue and Longevity for the proper ratio and optimum dosage).
- Avoid stimulants such as caffeine, alcohol, tobacco, soda, sugar and excessive carbohydrates.
- Supplements that are very beneficial include antioxidants, EFAs, vitamin C, E, and all B vitamins, magnesium (alone or coupled with calcium), and zinc (with 2 mg of copper).
- Raw vegetable juice (For my personal formula, refer to the Initial Protocol in Chapter 5).
- Adaptogenic herbs such as ginseng, rhodiola and ashwagandha
- Bee pollen and propolis

- Algae, including blue-green and chlorella
- Amino acid complex
- Pregnenolone: Sources are available from Source Naturals, Life Extension, Nutri Meds, Swanson Vitamins, Only Natural, Country Life, Douglas Laboratories. Natures Plus, Vitacost, Natural Balance
- DHEA Sources are available from Natures Plus, Life Extension, Vitamin Shoppe Brand, Douglas Laboratories
- Phosphytidylserine: useful for both underactive and overactive adrenal dysfunction. This component is hailed for its ability to lower cortisol. It is suggested for both overactive and underactive because of its impressive effect upon the hypothalamus gland. The hypothalamus happens to be a key regulator between the adrenal glands and the pituitary gland. Sources are available from Natural Factors, Natures Way, Natures Plus, Source Naturals, Doctor's Best, Jarrow Formulas, Now Foods, Solgar, Sangsters, and Vitamin Shoppe.
- L-Tyroisne is also earmarked for the adrenal glands. The two main adrenal hormones, epinephrine and adrenaline, are formed from the amino acid tyrosine.

CHAPTER THREE

Past, Present and Future Direction of Bowel Disorders

"What the patient takes beyond his ability
to digest does harm."

—Gee, S. 1888

History of Inflammatory Bowel Disorders (IBD)

Historical accounts reveal that in 300 BCE, a Roman physician described in detail symptoms of diarrhea resembling those of celiac disease. Insinuations of fasting were reported along, with the use of juice from the plantain plant, a member of the banana family, shown to cure the disease. Another report in medical literature took place in 1745, describing how Prince Charles had a medical condition, ulcerative colitis, and was said to have cured himself by adopting a milk-free diet.[1]

During the 1980s, Dr. von Brandes and Dr. Lorenz-Meyer of Marburg, West Germany, conducted a randomized study involving a treatment for Crohn's disease. The trial consisted of 20 participants with Crohn's disease symptoms who underwent a diet which excluded any refined carbohydrates and sugar substances. The subjects experienced remission of their symptoms. Another similar study by a group of doctors in 1985 involved the premise of "maintenance of remission by diet," implementing the elimination of certain foods; in particular, dairy products and cereals. The

---

1   deDombal, F.T.1968, Postgraduate Medical Journal 44:684-692

results of this study were sustained remissions. The physicians carrying out this research stated that "dietary manipulation might be an effective long term therapeutic strategy for Crohn's disease."

Dr. Heaton, author of a paper on the subject of inflammatory bowel disease, reported that all studies found sucrose intake to be higher in Crohn's patients than in people without Crohn's disease. Dr. Heaton reports, "The consistency of this finding is remarkable considering the variety of countries and methods used to carry out the studies. Among the patients in the seventeen studies reported, found that sucrose intake varied from between 20 percent to 220 percent more in Crohn's patients than in people who did not develop Crohn's disease. In conclusion, the connection between Crohn's disease and a sugar rich diet is proved beyond a reasonable doubt. Apart from smoking, this is the strongest clue to an environmental etiology of the disease."[2]

A physician and professor from Columbia University, Dr. Herter made the observation that in every case where children were wasting away from diarrhea and impairment, proteins were favorably endured, fats were managed fairly well, but carbohydrates, sugars and starches were adversely tolerated. He stated that, "Ingestion of some carbohydrates almost inevitably produced a relapse or a return of diarrhea after a period of improvement."[3]

During a similar time, Dr. Samuel Gee, who specialized in children's care, evidently noticed a recurrence of symptoms that continue to be ignored by many modern day specialists. Dr. Gee stated, "If the patient with intestinal disease could be cured at all, it would have to be by means of diet." He added that milk was the least suitable food during intestinal problems and that extremely starchy food like rice, corn, potatoes or grains were unfit. Dr. Gee continued, "We must never forget that what the patient takes, beyond his power to digest, does harm."

Be aware that, in cases of digestive disorders or compromised assimilation, all foods taken in should require minimal digestion, especially carbohydrates. Undigested carbohydrate will not be absorbed. These unabsorbed carbohydrates are not departing benignly through the small intestine and colon to be eliminated, but ultimately travel elsewhere in the digestive tract causing problems, all the while providing a smorgasbord for the microbial population.

2   Heaton, K.W. 1990. Inflammatory Bowel Diseases, Eds. R.N. Allan, M.R.B. Keighley; Churchill Livingstone, New York.
3   Herter, C. (1910), Transactions of the Association of American Physicians 25:528.

Frequent Characteristics of IBD

- Crohn's disease, ulcerative colitis, celiac, and irritable bowel syndrome (IBS) have repeatedly been linked with lactose and gluten intolerances.
- Even though colitis is normally relegated to the large colon, there are times when a so-called backwash ileitis may develop, advancing into the small intestine.
- Patients with IBS, Crohn's, colitis and celiac disease ate corn flakes more frequently than the general public. Since corn is gluten-free, people feel it is a grain substitute. Regrettably, corn is a known allergen and also has mycotoxins, a fungus.
- People with severe gut symptoms have an increased risk for malnutrition.
- Other problems that may have an affiliation with gut disorders include psychological disorders, arthritis, blood clots, lower immune response, eye infections, liver disease, gallstones and skin problems.
- Food allergies can also develop as a result of damage to the surface of the small intestine.
- Leaky gut syndrome is closely associated with the development of allergies and malabsorption problems.

General Risk Factors of IBD

- Family history of gastrointestinal complaints
- Traditional diet including high starch and sugar content
- Consumption of a high fat diet especially from dairy and meat products
- Sick often/vulnerable to illnesses
- Frequent diarrhea, blood in stool
- Discomfort after eating—gas, belching, bloated feeling, indigestion
- Stress, worry, unhappiness
- Lethargy
- Weight loss
- Crohn's and colitis are both associated with an increased frequency of colon cancer.
- All gut dysbiosis conditions have a chance to interfere with the normal efforts of the body to restore health.

- Prolonged usage of medications: anti-inflammatory, antibiotics, pain and some anti-depressants
- Risk of surgery: Portions of the colon removed, or a permanent procedure such as colostomy. Colostomy is a surgical process where a portion of the colon is brought through the abdomen wall, thus bypassing normal bowel evacuation. A bag is applied to the area to collect the fecal matter and protect the clothing. This operation may be temporary or permanent. It often accompanies procedures involving the removal of the large colon.

Medications Prescribed for Gastrointestinal Complaints

- Entyvio is one of the newest drugs being recommended for patients who do not respond favorably to corticosteroids, immunomodulators, or tumors necrosis factor blocker medications.
- Humira (adalimumab) is an injectable protein (antibody) being used to treat various forms of inflammation for arthritic conditions, Crohn's and other similar complaints.
- Imuran (azathioprine) is described as a chronic immunosuppressant antimetabolite drug, often recommended for Crohn's disease and colitis.
- Prednisone is classified as a corticosteroid drug. It is routinely used as an anti-inflammatory and immunosuppressive treatment for chronic allergic reactions involving swelling and itching; systemic lupus, rheumatoid arthritis, blood diseases, nausea and vomiting, various kidney diseases, brain edema and so on.
- Sulfasalazine is the most common drug prescribed for IBD. Sulfasalazine's bioavailability consists of one third of its dosage being absorbed from the small intestine while the remaining two-thirds passes into the colon.
- Mesalamine: When sulphasalazine is not tolerated, you may be put on mesalamine drugs, generally known as S-ASA agents.
- Corticosteroids are often prescribed for inflammation, but cause serious side effects including greater susceptibility to infection.

- 6-mercaptopurine and the related drug azathioprine are immune-suppressing drugs. They work by blocking the immune reaction that contributes to inflammation.
- Remicade is used for the treatment of moderate to severe Crohn's that does not respond to mesalamine substances, corticosteroids, immunosuppressive drugs and is used for treatment of open, draining fistulas.
- Infliximab has an anti-tumor or necrosis factor (TNF) substance. TNF is a protein produced by the immune system. Anti-TNF removes the TNF from the bloodstream before it reaches the intestines, thereby preventing inflammation.
- Antibiotics, which treat bacterial infection.
- Budersonide is a new corticosteroid that appears to be as effective as other corticosteroids but causes fewer side effects.
- Methotexate and cyclosporine are immunosuppressive drugs that may be useful. They appear to work faster than traditional immunosuppressive drugs.
- Natalizumab is an experimental drug that decreases inflammation by binding to immune cells.

Consumers and health care professionals are encouraged to report adverse reactions from the use of Entyvio or Azathioprine to the FDA's MedWatch Adverse Event Reporting program at www.fda.gov/MedWatch or by calling 1-800-FDA-1088.

Carbohydrate Breakdown

Carbohydrates, above all other food groups, hold the greatest influence over intestinal microbes throughout the process of fermentation. The word "carbohydrate" refers to starch and disaccharide sugar molecules, both of which require digestion before they can be absorbed by the body. Malabsorption refers to the inability of our body cells to obtain nutrients from the foods we eat.

The carbohydrates found in fruit, honey, yogurt and certain vegetables are single sugars. Glucose, for example, is a single sugar molecule, biochemically referred to as a monosaccharide. It is a predigested sugar, which means it is a food source readily available to the body. A disaccharide describes two sugar molecules, such as table sugar and sucrose. A polysaccharide is a starch consisting of multiple sugar molecules.

Microbes require energy for continued maintenance and growth, which they obtain from the fermentation of available carbohydrates that remain in the intestinal tract. Unabsorbed carbohydrates are the major source of gas in the intestines. For instance, the lactose contained in one ounce of milk, if undigested and unabsorbed, will manufacture about 50 ml of gas in the intestine of an average person (although, when intestinal microbes invade the small intestine under unstable conditions, the production of hydrogen gas may escalate to over one hundred fold).

The undigested carbohydrates within the small intestine can also impact the microbes in the colon. When the rate of undigested carbohydrates entering the large colon accelerates, so too does the proliferation of micro-bacterium. These higher-than-normal levels of bacteria will seep into the small intestine, where they will establish themselves and further multiply.

Lactic, acetic and other short chain organic acids, along with gas, can injure the small intestine. In conjunction with the damage to the intestine from microbial sources, research has revealed supporting evidence that lactic acid formed from fermentation in the intestine may be a contributing factor in abnormal brain function and behavior. These studies also help to explain the behavioral problems which often accompany intestinal disorders.

The fermentation of unabsorbed carbohydrates influences the growth of large quantities of lactic acid. Consequently, we see a continuance of malabsorption within the gut which can only extend the complaint or condition. This may be prevented by following a diet which restricts certain carbohydrates.

In addition to this intimidating cycle, the bacterial growth in the small intestine encourages the destruction of enzymes on the intestinal cell walls, inhibiting carbohydrate digestion and absorption. The increased availability of carbohydrates for further fermentation leads to the production of excessive mucus (which may be the consequence of a self defense device by the body). The intestinal surface then increases mucus production in an attempt to protect itself against injury with lubrication, a process initiated by microbial toxins, acids and the presence of partially digested and unassimilated carbohydrates.

The goal of a controlled carbohydrate diet is to nourish the individual while decreasing or otherwise cutting off the food supply to the harmful intestinal bacteria. The restriction of certain carbohydrates assists in the reduction and altering of bacterial growth, while providing an optimum state of health for the individual. With the reduction of intestinal microbes, stress on the intestine decreases, allowing those carbohydrates requiring minimal digestion to be absorbed, essentially leaving no carbs behind to further procreate bacteria in the intestine.

Once the body no longer requires protection from harmful bacteria, the production of mucus is reduced and carbohydrate assimilation is improved, replacing malabsorption with absorption. All the cells of the body resume being fed, including the immune system, which is instrumental in conquering microbial assault.

The standard Western diet is high in fats, carbohydrates and highly processed foods with many additives and preservatives, and is the root cause of many digestive disorders. According to Patrick Donvan, N.D., there are many causes of gastrointestinal disorders, including dietary and nutritional factors, food allergies, viral and bacterial infections, parasites, and stress. He states, "They can also be secondary to problems with the pancreas, liver or gallbladder, all of which are involved in the digestive process." Dr. Donovan continues, "Many of these disorders involve inflammation of part of the digestive tract, which may be secondary to any of the above causes." Disturbance of the digestive system can lead to malabsorption and nutritional deficiencies.

How to Avoid Chronic Gastrointestinal Illness
When seeking to avoid chronic gastrointestinal illness, early detection will help in many cases. However, lifestyle changes, particularly a change in diet, will produce the quickest reversal and healing of intestinal ailments. Become familiar with the problems of over-medicating and the intake of strong dosages of antibiotics and anti-inflammatory drugs that routinely cause intestinal inflammation. Many suggestions for symptoms associated with gut dysbiosis and other complaints are included throughout this book. Correcting nutritional deficiencies through dietary means and additional supplementation is preferable as a curative measure, especially when one's daily diet is not providing all the essential nutrients required for a full disease reversal and continued health maintenance. We *can* stop the further weakening the body and its systems by eliminating harmful substances such as coffee, junk food and the many items listed in the various diet segments throughout this publication. Don't worry; many of these will be temporary—just until sufficient healing has taken place.

Diarrhea Overview

Diarrhea is described as frequent bowel movements, accompanied by liquid or very soft feces. Prolonged or chronic diarrhea promotes loss of vital salts and nutrients. Diarrhea is another of the body's ways to rapidly eliminate germs, toxins, and irritants from the gastrointestinal tract. Diarrhea results in dehydration, excessive loss of fluids and loss of potassium and electrolytes. This condition is often associated with other digestive system disorders, such as colitis, Crohn's disease, celiac and irritable bowel syndrome. People often suffer with diarrhea when they are lactose intolerant, have food allergies, drink contaminated water, suffered food poisoning, bacterial infection and other causes. If a person has a history of diarrhea or rectal discharge, a sigmoidoscopy or MRI scan may be recommended to determine whether more degenerative conditions such as Crohn's disease or colitis are present. Recently, MRI scans have started being recommended more often, as they are a less invasive option which does not cause irritation to the already compromised tissue; it may also provide extra information.

A colonoscopy and a sigmoidoscopy are diagnostic procedures used to check for cancer and polyps. A colonoscopy is typically used for checking the whole colon, whereas a sigmoidoscopy is for investigating the lower portion of the colon. A sigmoidoscopy procedure utilizes a sigmoidoscope or illuminated tube, which passes through the anus into the rectum and sigmoid colon, revealing the diseased mucous membrane. To examine the upper regions of the colon, a barium enema would be performed.

Constipation Overview

Constipation occurs when fecal matter stagnates, causing pain, gas and bloating. The feces typically become hard and compacted, creating difficult evacuation. Constipation can result from low intake of fiber and fluids, inappropriate diet, not answering nature's call and inadequate exercise. Unfortunately, many people have also inherited sluggish or lazy colons, and most likely have a history of this complaint for almost as long as they can remember.

The bowels function best when the body is devoid of stress and anxiety—in other words, a relaxed state. Side effects from iron and inappropriate use of laxatives, along with certain drugs such as pain killers and antidepressants can promote constipation. The Western diet is notoriously too high in overcooked food and refined starches that leave a mushy, paste-like consistency in the bowels. A healthy colon requires adequate fiber and water for peristaltic action to take place effectively.

Laxatives are irritants which stimulate the bowels, causing it to work constantly, often resulting in structural damage to the colon. The bowels become dependent on such irritants, producing an undesirable opposite effect—a loss of muscle tone, which ultimately promotes a weakness in that muscle structure. Longterm use and dependency on laxative substances will permanently destroy the ability of the bowel to eliminate normally. I have even witnessed the anus walls sliding out upon pressure from the individual trying to eliminate, due to the inappropriate and extended use of laxative drug medication. Whether you are using a natural herbal laxative or medication, prolonged use of such substances will equate to the same, in the weakening and damage of intestinal tissue integrity.

Keep in mind that the frequency or quantity of fecal elimination is not an indication as to the absence of constipation in the bowels. A person can have several small movements a day and still be constipated. There is also such an occurrence as "over flow" a term being popularized today which describes an impacted colon, and yet the patient has symptoms of diarrhea.

What Does Healthy Stool (Fecal Matter) Look Like?
Ideally, your fecal matter should be lighter in color, more appropriately yellowish brown or light brown, with a smooth texture, floating near the surface in water. The color is a gauge (more or less) of the bacterial environment in your large colon. The lighter the color, the more good bacteria exists there. If the color of your stool is dark brown or similar in shade and ball-shaped, your friendly flora is low, and you are constipated even if you eliminate everyday. Regardless of daily defecation, the labeling of constipation still holds, because it takes considerable compacting of fecal matter within the colon to form the ball shapes and hardness of the mass when one defecates (which may resemble the colon itself).

Dr. Bernard Jensen, a well-known nutritionist, had sent fecal samples from 500 of his patients to a medical laboratory to find out all he could about their intestinal flora. The lab results averaged a ratio of 85 percent *bacillus coli* (or detrimental bacteria) in comparison to 15 percent *acidophilus* (the opposite of what the ratio should be). Dr. Jensen recommends taking care of constipation through colonics, a cleansing process. He advocates that a real cleansing process should be one that reaches every cell in the body. In the same vein, I also recommend addressing the lymph system, which is an important area to keep clean and maintained. In general, we can say that the blood is only as clean as the bowels; since blood circulates through every organ in the body and reaches every cell in the body, toxins in the blood due to an unclean bowel may contaminate the entire body. To properly cleanse the body tissue, we must start with a thorough cleansing of the bowels and continue on to the rest of the body.

Most of the nutrients from our food are passed through the intestinal wall of the small intestine. Poor assimilation leads to nutritional deficiencies. It is not only what we eat, it is what we absorb that counts. Digestion will not be optimum in a toxic body. Poisons such as tobacco, coffee, alcohol, chocolate, medications, and sugar have detrimental effects on our elimination and digestion processes. Toxins and unwanted substances find their way to all parts of our body via the lymph and blood vessels. Your fat tissue is also a place where toxins get stored en masse. Lose weight, and you will have a cleaner body.

Diverticulosis and Diverticulitis Overview

Diverticular disease consists of a spectrum of conditions whose symptom awareness can range from acute to chronic diverticulitis. The presence of diverticula within the colon indicates diverticulosis, while diverticulitis consists of inflammation of a diverticulum. Note that diverticular disease can also exist symptom-free.

Constipation is directly linked to diverticular disease, and heads the list of many concerns, due to low fiber intake. There are also many other physical problems that materialize from a low fiber diet.

Dr. Dennis Burkitt of London, England is recognized for his investigative work and innovative application of fiber in the diet. He states, "There is now a fairly well-defined list of diseases that are recognized as characteristic of modern Western culture. All of them have their minimum presence in economically more developed countries and are rare in rural communities in the Third World. These diseases include ischemic heart disease, gallstones, diabetes, obesity, varicose veins, deep vein thrombosis, hiatus hernia, colorectal cancer, appendicitis, diverticular disease, and hemorrhoids. There is evidence to suggest that all the diseases in this list are diet related. The reduction in intake of dietary fiber and in cereal fiber in particular, is the diet change that has been predominately incriminated in the increased prevalence of certain gastrointestinal diseases, in Western countries mainly, during the past half century."[4]

Regular Bowel Movements Prevent Diverticulosis
Diverticulitis is classified as a civilized disease and is commonly seen in nearly half the population over the age of 50. This disorder has become very common in Western countries, but is rarely seen in parts of the world such as Africa, where a high fiber diet is standard. North America and England may top the list for this condition, although other industrialized countries have adopted a similar lifestyle of ingesting far too many refined carbohydrates containing white flour, sugar and other low fiber foods.

Diverticulosis occurs when the mucous lining of the muscle wall of the intestines protrudes out forming sac-like pouches (diverticulum). Once these pouches become inflamed, due to small particles of food becoming lodged in the pouches, the patient develops diverticulitis. Although diverticuli may occur anywhere in the digestive tract, they typically occur towards the end of the large intestine/sigmoid colon region and may be present in the descending colon. These conditions are far easier to prevent than to treat.

In 2007, The World Gastroenterology Organization reported an estimated 25 percent of diverticular cases had complications with abscesses, fistula, obstruction, peritonitis, and sepsis. Compiled studies gave much insight into the age categories affecting individuals with diverticular disease:

PREVALENCE BY AGE	PREVALENCE BY GENDER
Age 40: 5 percent	Age 50: more common in males
Age 60: 30 percent	Age 60: more common in males
Age 80: 65 percent	Age 70: more common in women

The statistics show that diverticuli are present in about 25 percent of men and an excess of 50 percent of women. Approximately 200,000 persons or more are hospitalized each year in the United States alone with diverticulitis. An impacted bowel can lead to the severe problem of colon cancer. Regular bowel movements will prevent serious illnesses of the colon such as these. Not surprisingly, diverticular disease is far less common in vegetarians. It is generally agreed upon that not only will a high fiber diet *prevent* the forma-

---

4   "Fiber as Protective Against Gastrointestinal Diseases," Dennis Burkitt, C.M.G., F.R.S., M.D., F.R.C.S., Back to Eden, Jethro Kloss, (1994), 570-578.

tion of diverticuli, but it will also *improve* the symptoms of diverticulosis that are currently present. (Refer to Chapters 5 and 13 for more information on fiber, and Chapter 12 for more information on constipation.)

Irritable Bowel Syndrome (IBS) Overview

Irritable bowel syndrome is yet another modern day disorder, one which afflicts over 220 million people worldwide. Irritable bowel syndrome is a disorder of the intestines reported to affect 20 percent of the population, or one in five adults. These people either already have these symptoms or will experience them sometime in their life. Spastic colitis, mucous colitis, nervous stomach, nervous diarrhea, spastic colon, or functional bowel disease are all references and common names of IBS. The term most frequently used today is irritable bowel syndrome. Regardless of the name, suffering from this symptomatic disorder is debilitating and lifestyle restricting. Irritable bowel syndrome should not be confused with inflammatory bowel diseases like Crohn's disease, ulcerative colitis or celiac.

A partial list of warning signs for IBS includes the following: fever, weight loss, painful or difficult swallowing, continual vomiting and feeling full sooner than normal during meals. Diarrhea or a change in bowel configuration, such as worsening constipation, narrowing stools or blood in the stool may be other signs. Holistic treatment of IBS involves the use of natural alternative remedies, consisting of various traditional herbal medicines for the relief of abdominal pain, bloating, diarrhea, constipation and anxiety.

A primary symptom of IBS is either persistent or recurring abdominal gas pain. The consequence of gas pain is often accompanied with embarrassing symptoms of sudden, unexpected spells of diarrhea, belching and excessive gas. Sporadic or chronic constipation is also common. People with the medical condition irritable bowel syndrome are rarely regular; their bowel movements are inclined to be either too fast or too slow. Acquainting oneself with the location of the rest room when out and about becomes a way of life for people with IBS or spastic colon. The fear of not having sufficient time to get to the facilities is enough to trigger symptoms and discourage attendance at many social functions. Accessibility and availability of rest rooms becomes a vital concern in life.

There is no exclusive profile for a person with irritable bowel syndrome. People from all different professions and gender can be affected. Factors causing irritable bowel may be psychological, physical or a combination of both. The exact cause of IBS is still unknown; it is understood *what* happens, but not completely *why*. Emotional stress or physical factors such as food sensitivities must be investigated to determine the cause of this bothersome condition. Irritable bowel syndrome could even have a hereditary predisposition. Evidence to watch for would be recurrent abdominal pain during childhood which may indicate a predisposition to the development of this disorder.

The antibiotic Metronidazole, used to treat infections of the urinary and digestive systems, often triggers irritable bowel symptoms. Antibiotics are known generators for candidiasis (yeast infections). Practitioners of alternative medicine have suggested that colonization of the gastrointestinal tract with yeasts may result in irritable bowel syndrome. If the gut has insufficient levels of its beneficial bacteria, (*lactobacillus acidophilus* and *bifidus*) the resident yeasts are not likely to multiply. Once the yeasts have overgrown to excess in the digestive system, they will ferment food, in particular, sugar—producing alcohol and alcohol breakdown products. In order to avoid this condition, recolonization of normal bacteria with probiotic supplementation, yogurt, kefir, clabbered milk or similar types of products along with a diet free of yeast and/or sugar is recommended.

Many professionals have characterized irritable bowel syndrome as not being a single disorder, but rather a spectrum of disorders resulting from inconsistencies at all levels of the gut. Proper nutrition for optimum health is always important but absolutely essential if you have IBS. Our bodies react automatically when we eat. Eating should be a pleasurable experience, but for anyone suffering from irritable bowel syndrome, it is clouded with apprehension as to when and what symptoms may arise.

Treatment for irritable bowel syndrome, as with other intestinal disorders, begins with education. Every person's system is different and reacts uniquely. A variety of causes will provoke symptoms. Stress leads to emotional diarrhea, as observed with "butterflies in the stomach." Concern often arises as to whether or not this condition will develop into colitis. But the word colitis imitates inflammation of the colon; irritable bowel syndrome is not affiliated with colon inflammation, and should not be misinterpreted with inflammatory bowel disease. Inflammatory bowel disease (IBD) patients will often have bloody diarrhea, fever, and symptoms of weight loss associated with colon inflammation. (Refer to Chapter 12 for treatment and diet plans.)

Celiac Disease Overview

Celiac disease is triggered by consumption of the plant protein gluten, which is found in grains like wheat, barley and rye. Currently, research is shedding light on the sequence of events which produce the T-cell antigens to specific polypeptides or hydrolysates of gluten. Other conditions related to gluten sensitivities are gluten ataxia and dermatitis herpetiformis. Further studies and education will hopefully pinpoint the amino acid sequence in the gluten protein of grasses.

As far back as 1908, doctors reported incidences of patients suffering with malabsorption and extended periods of diarrhea. They started witnessing deterioration of the brain and spinal cord, as well as other areas of the nervous system. These failing conditions were then, as now, attributed to malabsorption of vital nutrients due to a damaged intestinal tract. Evidence to support these theories started appearing throughout research papers as science advancements were made. Since then, many discoveries have been made helping to explain why so many reactions are occurring that are related to biological factors. Such findings include many types of mental disorders and physical disorders connected to yeast infections. Other areas of interest were studies on neurological disorders associated with adult celiac disease and psychoses with digestive origins.

Many of these studies involved measuring the level of toxins within the intestinal tract, which were affecting normal brain function and the overgrowth of intestinal microbes. In 1982 the New England Journal of Medicine reported on D-lactic acid, a waste product from bacterial fermentation, which was invading brain tissue and harming brain cells. Chronic diarrhea and epileptic seizure episodes were also occurring in babies. Once a child is weaned and put on formula or solid food, problems such as these began taking place. Favorable results were reported when certain grains and dairy products were removed from the diet. The protein gluten found in many grains and lactose in dairy are often times the offending substances promoting imbalances throughout the body of sensitive individuals.

In 2015, the American College of Gastroenterology reported the prevalence of celiac disease in the United States to be similar to that of other European countries, indicating 0.71 percent (or 1 in 141). Furthermore, an estimated 83 percent of Americans who have celiac disease are either misdiagnosed or undiagnosed. On a positive note, the National Foundation for Celiac Awareness has calculated based on public awareness that the celiac disease diagnosis rate could reach 50–60 percent by 2019.[5] Celiac patients show an increased risk of 30 percent to develop malignancy such as non-Hodgkin's lymphoma. With the many debilitating risks facing celiac patients, adhering to a gluten-free diet is critical for preventing further complications.

In Canada, the prevalence of celiac disease through research-based statistics is between 0.5–1 percent. When compared to the statistics in Europe, it is felt that this ratio is misrepresentative, and shows a much higher incidence of celiac. The most recent studies found celiac disease affected 1 in 100 Canadians, with the diagnosis rate increasing each year. Nearly 30 percent of Canadian children with celiac disease are initially misdiagnosed.

Unquestionably, this is a widespread problem requiring a great deal of attention, especially since most of these individuals remain undiagnosed. Fortunately, there are various medical centers and specialists covering unique aspects of celiac disease in children and infants. Early detection and management is vital for their continued health and happiness. It is possible to keep celiac disease under control by implementing a gluten-free diet. (Refer to Chapters 12 and 13 for safe grains/ingredients and news on the Government Gluten Alert Program.)

2011 Warren Prize in Celiac Disease

Frits Koning, Ph.D. is the recipient of the 2011 William K. Warren, Jr. Prize for Excellence in Celiac Disease Research. He is head of the Immunochemistry Section in the Department of Immunohematology and Blood Transfusion of the Leiden University Medical Centre (LUMC), the Netherlands. The award was presented by Mr. William K. Warren Jr. Professor Koning gave the 2011 Warren Prize Lecture, "Celiac Disease: How Complicated Can It Get?" on June 3, 2011.

Other Past Award Recipients of the Warren Prize in Celiac Disease Studies:

2010: Bana Jabri, M.D., Ph.D., University of Chicago
Markku Mäki, M.D., Ph.D., University of Tampere, Finland
2008: Salvatore Auricchio, M.D., Ph.D., University "Federico II," Naples, Italy
2007: Ludvig M. Sollid, M.D., Ph.D., Institute of Immunology, University of Oslo

---

5 Datamonitor Group, 2015

Crohn's Disease/Ulcerative Colitis (Pancolitis) Overview

In 1932, Dr. B.B. Crohn lectured on a new intestinal disorder, which he called regional ileitis (and which is now known as Crohn's disease). Crohn's disease and ulcerative colitis are both chronic inflammatory intestinal conditions. The difference between the two is mainly the location and the degree of degeneration in the intestinal mucosal tissue. Ulcerative colitis is normally regulated to the colon and rectum, whereas Crohn's disease may affect any segment of the alimentary canal, from the esophagus to the anus (but more commonly affects the last portion of the small intestine, referred to as the ileum). Crohn's disease of the small intestine is also known as regional enteritis, while involvement of the colon is properly referred to as Crohn's disease, or granulomatous colitis.

Crohn's disease has increased in incidence since its discovery in 1932, not only in Western society but also in third world populations. It occurs about equally in both sexes, race and age throughout the world. Unfortunately, colitis and Crohn's disease complaints are also associated with an increased frequency of colonic cancer. Colon cancer is very common, with more than 120,000 new cases diagnosed in North America each year. That number has been on the rise (as has all incidences of cancer). Mainstream research is not showing any specific genetic link of inherent weakness or genetic predisposition to inflammatory bowel diseases. Although bowel inflammation is two to five times more common in Caucasians than in non-Caucasians, it is four times more common in Jewish heritage than in non-Jewish. In addition, multiple members of a family having Crohn's disease or ulcerative colitis make up between 15–40 percent of cases.

Dr. Andrew R. M.D. at Cooper University Hospital reported estimates on Crohn's Disease in United States and Canada. Dr. Andrew and the Genetic Counseling Staff reported that approximately 630,000 individuals suffer from Crohn's disease, and between 10,000 and 47,000 are diagnosed every year throughout both countries.[6] Ulcerative colitis has recently been renamed pancolitis. It is not unlike Crohn's disease in that its symptoms affect 50 out of every 100,000 people in the United States. Most cases of ulcerative colitis develop between the ages of 15 and 35, although children and older adults also develop the disease. The majority of cases diagnosed with ulcerative colitis are aged 20 or older.

---

6 Loftus EV. Clinical epidemiology of inflammatory bowel disease: incidence, prevalence, and environmental influences. Gastro.2004;126 (6):1504–17.

Collagenous colitis, by contrast, is lighter in symptoms compared to pancoliltis or the more typical colitis complaints. Collagenous colitis is covered in its entirety in Chapter 12, including a full treatment plan, causes, and related symptoms.

Many attempts have been made to verify a bacterial, mycobacterium, fungal or viral origin as responsible for intestinal disorders. Mental and physical considerations, such as psychosomatic illness, stress, and emotional trauma may play an important role as a contributing factor in advancing the disease. One of my former patients developed colitis from overwork and emotional stress. When their lifestyle eventually settled down, their condition systemically went away. It has been several years now, and still no symptoms, but a case history such as this has not been commonplace. (Refer to the Initial Protocol in Chapter 5.)

The initial cause of Crohn's disease is not a single entity, but is rather viewed as many disturbances which often seem to be the result of auto-immune disorders or food allergies. To assist in diagnosing this problem, x-rays are taken of the terminal ileum, a customary location, looking for abnormalities. A few stressful and painful symptoms include diarrhea, flatulence, abdominal tenderness, fever, anorexia and weight loss and a general feeling of being in poor health. Holistic treatment includes a wide variety of natural health applications to address the many different aspects of an inflammatory bowel disorder.

CHAPTER FOUR

Holistic Approach for Certain Intestinal Disease Complications

About Type 'A' Crohn's Disease and Chronic Crohn's Disease Patients

Determining the range of severity in a case of Crohn's disease depends on many factors, such as how limiting or restrictive their diet needs to be in order to reach a full recovery. In addition to the specifics of their diet program, how many complaints need to be addressed? During an assessment, a person's symptoms will be used to determine the type of disorder they actually have, and to what degree of seriousness. The patient's symptoms are an important component in determining their actual condition (unless a medical procedure diagnosed otherwise). For example, patients have come to me complaining of Crohn's disease, when in actuality they were suffering from irritable bowel syndrome.

A classic type 'A' patient is usually unable to digest carbohydrates, which equates to not being able to digest certain sugars in the small intestine. Essentially, when a person cannot break down the sugars in some foods, those particles become a significant food supply for the millions of microbes in our gut. The microbial population becomes so prolific that they can damage the colon wall, sometimes to the point of decaying it, at which point surgery is required to remove the decayed tissue.

The holistic approach in cases such as these has the prevention of surgery as its primary goal. Initially, all factors that compromise the immune's systems defense would be addressed, and the microbe's food supply drastically diminished through dietary means. The body is thus brought back to a more balanced state by correcting the many nutritional deficiencies,

43

with the application of non-drug solutions for symptom complaints. On a positive note, we know that the cells in the intestines are the fastest at self-replicating—given time, the entire gut may be replaced. By reducing harmful bacteria in the gut, a person can stop breaking their body down, all the while enhancing the healing process.

Patients who suffer with serious Crohn's complaints typically lead a very poor quality of life. Their condition progressively gets worse, while their bowels are degenerating to the point where doctors are required to perform surgery and remove parts of, or even the entire large colon. Obtaining treatment through allopathic medicine will remedy symptoms such as bleeding, pain and gas, but the cause will not be addressed (as with most gastrointestinal disorders). In all fairness to these specialists, if a patient is not seeing them regularly for medications or requiring surgery, their job would be considerably easier.

There are certain disorders—such as gut dysbiosis and allergies, for instance—where allopathic medicine is ineffective in patients looking to attain overall full recovery *without* continuing medications. If only medications could cure the problem! But in these particular types of illnesses, the success rates are very low. Typically, sufficient time and/or effort are not given to finding the causes; thus, treatment for the symptoms becomes the only option. To a large degree, by the time alternative professionals see the patients that we do, their condition is far progressed. They often appear to be in a state of hopelessness at ever getting well, since their illness continues to persist. But it is amazing how much improvement can be accomplished in a short amount of time. With the right amount of effort applied on their part, along with the proper guidance and nutritionally sound advice, patients *can* become well again.

Leaky Gut Syndrome is Associated with Most Gut Dysbiosis

Individuals with leaky gut syndrome do not absorb nutrients properly. A person's gut which has experienced a lot of inflammation and irritation from a variety of causes will usually have holes in it. There are a number of causes which can lead to damage and deterioration of the gut's mucosal barrier. A few of these include chemical toxicity, excessive alcohol consumption, chronic stress, infections, medications, lack of digestive enzymes, food intolerances, allergies, and nutritional deficiencies. Then we have conditions associated with leaky gut syndrome, such as gastric complaints, digestive disorders involving bloating, constipation and diarrhea as well as candidia and fungal infections.

Some professionals say that those of us who drink harsh stimulants like coffee, soda or alcohol have holes in our guts. Nevertheless, when a gut becomes damaged from extended periods of irritation, as seen in the cases of gut disorders, the intestinal lining will be far more permeable than a gut would be from a normal bad habit, such as too much coffee. The problem with this scenario is that substances like gluten (the protein found in grains) will slip *through* these holes and into the blood stream. The body does not tolerate this protein in the blood and instructs the immune system to remove it.

As many people know from taking too many antibiotics, once an invader has been recognized, the body will be on the alert for the next time it shows up. Consequently, a person who did *not* have a problem eating starches with gluten in the past *now* discovers an allergy or intolerance to the protein gluten. This condition may not be permanent, especially if the individual does not have a history of gluten intolerance. But the initial protocol will be the same (though the lucky ones may return to eating gluten products once the gut has been well healed).

For example, a person may have Crohn's disease and not be Type 'A,' and will therefore be able to return some, if not most of the "forbidden foods" back into their diet. In such cases, any offending food or substance would need to be reintroduced very slowly, to prevent triggering an immune response. Inflammation offers its own list of problems and deficiencies, as seen in the following information.

Nutritional Recommendations

Leaky gut syndrome is well known for producing a long list of mineral deficiencies, such as magnesium, zinc, calcium, boron, silicon and manganese. L-Glutamine assists in the protection of the mucous lining of the intestines and stomach. Other lost nutrients to be considered for supplementation are coenzyme Q10, B complex vitamins (especially folic acid and vitamin B12), and selenium. The occurrence of malabsorption is initiated by inflammation and results when the transporter of proteins in the gastrointestinal tract has been damaged and is no longer able to carry minerals from the intestine to the bloodstream. An example is the mineral magnesium; even with higher levels of supplementation, when the carrier protein for this mineral is damaged, an intake of higher dosages will not compensate. Take care to replenish magnesium, since metabolic systems require magnesium to function. Similarly a zinc deficiency—a necessary component for the immune system—produces its own list of problems, such as hair loss or baldness, and may also lead to high blood pressure and high cholesterol.

Dampening inflammation response in the body initally requires adequate omega 3 fatty acids. These fats are a necessary element to ensure a beneficial outcome. To further assist the gut in reducing the damaging effects of inflammation, the following dietary additions have proven to be of great value: additional antioxidant supplements will prevent tissue damage brought on by inflammation. To naturally increase antioxidant levels, include foods that contain high amounts of carotenoids found in carrots, squash and yams and berries. Exotic berries, such as acai, aronia, and wolfberry have extraordinary amounts of antioxidants, as do certain plant enzymes such as those found in green kamut, barley green, and whole leaf aloe vera juice with high MPS (muscopolysaccharide) content. Bioflavonoids, available in many foods including citrus fruits, onions, garlic, peppers, buckwheat, and black currants, are also useful. Other potent enhancements are spirulina, chlorella, bee pollen and royal jelly which all aid in the repair of leaky gut syndrome. A few more examples of staple supplements would be vitamin C and E, and amino acids like cysteine, N-acetyl-cysteine, methionine and reduced L-Glutathione, all of which are important antioxidants.

Another area of assistance to improve nutrient absorption is with substances equipped to aid the digestive process. Such items include the pancreatic enzyme, proteolytic enzymes like proteinase or serrapeptase, glutamic acid, hydrochloride, betaine hydrochloride, pepsin, apple cider vinegar, lemon juice and stomach bitters.

Lab Tests for Leaky Gut

This test will help determine how leaky your gut is. The test is called the lactulose-mannitol challenge test, which measures the permeability of the patient's gut. In performing this test, the patient consumes orally five grams each of the sugars lactulose and mannitol. The normal ratio within the gut is less than 1 percent permeable of lactulose, to approximately 14 percent of mannitol, which is a smaller molecule. Once absorbed, the test measures urinary excretion of both sugars and then compares the ratio of lactulose to mannitol. Under normal conditions, the gut would measure less than 0.03 percent of lacutlose to mannitol, whereas a leaky gut will register a higher ratio of lactulose to mannitol, indicating a loss of lactulose across the intestinal barrier wall.

Abscesses and Fistulas

A fistula is an opening that has been created between the anal canal and the surface of the skin. An abscess is inflamed tissue containing pus, usually caused by bacterial infection. Fistulas may develop after an abscess has broken in the rectum area. Underlying cause on several different levels often promotes abscesses, especially when they are recurring—problems with blood impurities, poor nutrition and a less than optimum immune system will greatly enhance a patient's susceptibility to abscesses and wounds not healing. For example, a person with an already inflamed rectum where tissue degeneration has commenced runs the risk of abscesses and fistulas developing internally, or in the external anal vicinity (as with conditions such as Crohn's disease and ulcerative colitis). Other, lesser intestinal disorders could also acquire this side effect, although it is primarily in severe gut disorders that abscesses and fistulas are more commonplace.

Nutrition Suggestions

Consider the term "clean diet." By that, I mean a diet which has removed all junk food, saturated fats, fried foods and pork. Foods such as these form toxic substances in the body that support infection and abscesses. The curative power of juicing is especially beneficial to assist a quicker healing process. (Refer to Chapters 5 and 9 for more information on juicing.) Eating a wide variety of colors, especially yellow and orange varieties of fruits and vegetables, is also of value. They are high in vitamin A, and serve as a natural laxative. Green vegetables rejuvenate the body by supporting the liver, blood and kidneys.

Recurring antibiotic usage often accompanies abscesses. To counter the harmful effects of antibiotics, eat adequate amounts of plain, unsweetened yogurt or other similar foods such as kefir, fermented red-beet juice or sauerkraut, ideally on a daily basis. Our friendly micro-flora is compromised by antibiotics, and these foods will help replenish and rebalance the beneficial bacteria within the gut.

Supplementation

- Zinc: From 30 mg up to 60 mg, with 3–4 mg copper. High doses of zinc over a protracted period can lead to a copper deficiency if copper is not available in the diet, or through some other supplement. Note that homes with copper piping provide adequate copper through the water supply.
- Vitamin C with bioflavonoids: 500–1000 mg, every few hours, or 3000 mg and up may be taken as long as the bowel is tolerant.
- Garlic: 4000 mg, or several fresh cloves should be eaten in food daily. Fresh garlic should only be heated through, to retain its healing properties—do not cook thoroughly.
- Lactobacillus acidophilus: Take 2 capsules twice a day, or 1 teaspoon of Bio-K or powder.
- Vitamin A: 25000 IU, up to 100000 IU in divided doses with food. This would preferably replaced (at least in part) with two to four cups of carrot juice.
- Beta-carotene (avoid during pregnancy), unless in fresh juice form.
- Vitamin E with mixed tocopherols: 400–800 IU. Vitamin E helps with scarring and has great antioxidant properties.
- Colloidal silver: This is at the top on my list for healing externally. It comes already conveniently prepared on bandages and Band-Aids. I also recommend taking colloidal silver internally to assist the immune system in destroying pathogens when applicable.
- Refer to "Natural Alternatives for Antibiotics and Destroying Superbugs" in Chapter 7 for more information on colloidal silver and other natural healing remedies.

Herbal Remedies

To treat abscesses and speed healing, make use of these helpful herbal remedies:

- Mix slippery elm powder with water to make a paste or gruel. For extra healing support, add a few drops of colloidal silver and eucalyptus oil to the water for anti-bacterial power. This can also be used in a hot poultice.

- When an abscess is draining and pus is at the center, apply a moist, warm to hot compress with gentle healing herbs such as chamomile, sage or thyme to soften and ripen the abscess.
- Aloe vera juice: Check for high muscopolysaccharide levels for quality content. Drink alone or in liquid, 2 ounce doses three or more times a day. Aloe vera gel can also be applied directly to skin infections if the tissue isn't too irritated. It contains astringent, natural antibiotic and analgesic properties.
- When an abscess has completely drained, apply Calendula salve or St. John's wort oil for soothing and a speedier recovery.
- Yarrow is another remedy that may be taken in tea form once the abscess has drained. It provides antiseptic, anti-inflammatory and astringent benefits. Add 1 cup boiling water to 1 teaspoon yarrow herb. Sip occasionally throughout the day.
- To aid the immune system in ridding the body of bacterial infection, take herbal anti-viral and anti-bacterial tincture formulas in liquid. Take 10–15 drops, three times a day (may also be consumed in tea form a few times a day). Look for combination formulas or make your own using echinacea, goldenseal and myrrh.
- Burdock has blood purifying properties which may be used in a poultice. In addition, burdock acts as an antibiotic and may be consumed as a tea or tincture a few times daily.
- Other poultice suggestions for abscesses include linseed flour, applied as hot as can be tolerated. Repeat once the abcess has cooled down, every few hours.
- Thoroughly cleanse abscesses twice daily with a clean cotton cloth soaked in a sage or chamomile infusion.
- Nettle and red clover teas or juices are excellent beverages for blood cleansing and promoting more rapid healing. Nettle is a nourishing herb often used as a tea for raising iron levels in the blood.
- Liquid chlorophyll: Add to water and drink a few times a day. Add two teaspoons to a glass of water (8–10 ounces). Do not heat.

Retention Enemas

Herbal and other natural remedies have great application in furthering the healing process of fistulas and abscesses. Refer to Chapter 11 for proper retention enema protocol.

Homeopathy

The word homeopathy is derived from the Greek word *homoios* and *pathos*, referring to similar and suffering. Homeopathic medicine involves dilutions of natural substances from plants, minerals and animals, to stimulate the body's natural healing response. The remedies are matched to symptoms or patterns based on the principle of "like cures like." Homeopathy has curative properties that, when used appropriately, helps remove boils and abscesses by stimulating the body's internal defense system. Homeopathy is symptom-specific, which means you must correlate your symptoms to the description of the remedy.

- Choose one remedy according to the symptom, using 6c strength. Place two tablets under the tongue and repeat four times daily until improvement is noticed.
- Consider the following for their benefits: Belladonna, Hepar sulphuris, Homeopathic Silicea

Other Suggestions

- Medicinal clay draws out impurities. Mix 1 tablespoon of clay in water to form a paste and apply fairly thick on abscesses. Cover with cotton gauze first, followed by a towel to secure in place. Repeat when dry. Once the abscess becomes ripe, the pustule opens and discharges pus, it may then be cleansed, at which point the healing process can begin.
- Do your best not to squeeze the boil, as the bacteria can lead to infection and slow down the healing process. Squeezing can also damage the subcutaneous tissue and form scars.

Topical Treatment
- Calendula ointment, zinc oxide cream, and/or vitamin A (squeezed out from a 10,000 IU capsule) can be applied

topically a few times a day. Another suggestion is to apply raw, unprocessed honey to the infected area locally on an external abscess, three times a day.

- Herbal Paste: Make a paste of goldenseal root powder and calendula succus (the juice of the marigold flower). Apply the formula over the abscess and leave it on for 12–24 hours. This preparation will help draw out the infection while encouraging the restoration of injured tissues.

- Slippery Elm Powder: Mix with hot water and make a cereal; you may add cinnamon for flavor. Benefits all bowel disorders and diarrhea. Also apply externally for abscesses, boils or ulcers

- Argimony: For bleeding and diarrhea, buy in tincture form and take 10–15 drops until bleeding subsides, or as recommended by a practitioner.

- Lady's Mantle is considered an excellent wound healer. It may be applied onto the fistula or abscess in a gauze soaked with cold tea or as a salve.

- Sources: Bach Flower Essence and Seroyal are also available through distributors like http://allcosmeticsource.com.

- Refer to Chapter 11 for more herbal product sources.

CHAPTER FIVE

Full Initiation of the Disease Reversal Process

Initial Protocol

Lack of Energy

One of the first symptoms my patients express when they meet me for the first time is, "I am tired" or "I have no energy." To a large degree an enervated body, or a body evidencing fatigue, owes their condition to the glands and organs of the endocrine system. Malabsorption and malnourishment are two other common problems with anyone suffering from Crohn's, colitis, celiac, irritable bowel syndrome and/or prolonged diarrhea. It is for this reason that the first step often entails the removal of known food related irritants and bad habits.

These food preparations are tailored to match the person's symptoms by way of tolerance. Initially this may involve very easy digestible meals, especially during persistent bouts of diarrhea or any other acute symptom of discomfort. Essentially, the healing process begins with doing one's best to stop the body from breaking down further.

Additional Contributing or Initiating Factors Other Than Food Related
The following questions are used to initiate a dialogue separate from diet-related causes or diet-continuance problems:

- Has the complaint been a problem for as long as you can remember?

- Did a significant event or problem take place within a year of developing your symptoms?
- Has there been an emotional event involving extreme heartache, either recently or in the past?
- In the past, was there a very strong antibiotic prescription taken or a prolonged usage of antibiotics?
- Is there any long term use of other medications in your history? If so, what?
- Have you been exposed to toxic chemicals through ingesting or inhaling? What is the source?
- Do you tend to be a worrier?
- Do you feel overwhelmed at any time?
- How are your coping skills?
- Would you classify yourself as being happy or unhappy? Explain?

The most important part of the patient's health history overview is what is being taken into the body and their food history, not only currently but also in the past. Once the symptoms are matched to certain foods or substances, an elimination diet commences. (An elimination diet consists of a restricted dietary program geared to reduce symptoms and contributing factors of the condition). From my experience, I will initially remove gluten from a patient's diet, mainly because most people's guts have some degree of leaky gut syndrome. (For more information on leaky gut syndrome, refer to Chapter 4). I also remove corn products: while corn does not have gluten, it *is* a known allergen. Additionally, corn often has an association with fungus, related to its processing or storage. Dairy is the third elimination, either in whole or in part, depending on each individual case history. Sugar is a contributing factor as well, feeding the micro-bacteria and reducing the immune system's efficacy.

Through conversation, many of the offending foods or substances in a person's diet can be determined. Explanation is given as to why these foods or substances promote the symptoms they do following their consumption. Food elimination also includes the removal of stimulants such as coffee, black tea, soda, alcohol, tobacco, and processed juices, drinks and food, as well as any other food item or substance that is currently not well-tolerated.

Coffee Must Be Taken Away
Coffee must be taken away until the gut has had a chance to heal over and calm down. Coffee is among the most irritating substances imaginable for the colon, as it is so highly acidic. Coffee is great as an enema, if the need presents itself, as a remedy for constipation. The general public often uses coffee in the morning as a laxative. Another issue with coffee is that the properties in the bean destroy the good flora in our gut. For those individuals who consume large amounts of coffee, a tip to lessen its harmful effects would be to chase it down with water for dilution and to flush it through the system more quickly.

Juicing Raw Vegetables and Fruit
Another tool I consistently use for restoring the body on many different levels is raw vegetable juicing. Vegetable juicing provides rapid healing when freshly made in its raw unprocessed state.

My first exposure to juicing was through a small paperback book written by Dr. Walker. He started extracting juice from plants using hydraulic presses in 1910. I once saw a picture of him in a magazine article, the title of which was something along the line of "In Praise of Carrot Juice." The picture was of Dr. Walker, age 109, holding a glass of carrot juice and looking not a day over 75. If you want to look young and feel younger, I highly recommend juicing.

Since one of the main problems for those with gut dysbosis is nourishing the body, the ease with which vegetable juice can be digested is very attractive. Consider the fine, hair like root fibers of a carrot, and imagine the minerals passing through those filaments; at this stage, the minerals have already been broken down within the carrot and are ready for assimilation. I myself have been juicing for more than thirty years, and make it a point to incorporate these liquids into my patients' healing therapy. Raw food in the form of juice is more readily absorbed and passes more easily through the gut wall. I am always fascinated to notice that, when I drink 20 ounces, I find that three hours has passed and I have yet to feel the need to answer the call of nature. This in and of itself speaks volumes to me as to how this liquid is being utilized in the body.

When putting a juice formula together to enhance health, it should feed as much of the body as possible, especially the blood, liver and kidneys. Other glands, like the thyroid and adrenal, will be supported directly with other supplements as detailed in Chapter 2. In the course of picking up the blood, all other areas of the body will start to respond favorably. The immune system will be boosted, promoting quicker healing of tissue. An increase of energy will be initially felt, and acidity will be lowered throughout the body. For these reasons and more, many people are coming to recognize how much better they feel and welcome juicing as part of their daily routine.

As a healing therapy, I recommend juicing once a day or more (based on individual determination). *Do not* substitute with processed store-bought varieties. You must make it yourself using a juicer and drink it within an hour. For a speedier recovery, juicing two or even three times a day will greatly enhance cellular regeneration.

Initially, to ensure bowel tolerance, adjustments may need to be implemented, such as fiber additives to firm up the feces and to slow down the number of bowel movements in a day. Also, consider the quantity of juice consumed at any given time. Drinking it slowly may be required. More guidance is provided in the Initial Quick Start Program included in this chapter.

Fresh juice is a food source that does not require energy from the body for digestion. If you are considering consuming raw juice more often, you will also prompt the body to cleanse toxins, wastes and chemicals throughout the entire body. Whereas, for maintenance of health, juicing five days a week will make an enormous difference in your life and longevity.

As a general rule, vegetables and fruits should not be combined into one juice formula (with exception to one apple per formula if a lighter, sweeter taste is desired). I suggest that, when looking to include fruit in one's diet, eating it as opposed to juicing it is preferable. Vegetables are high in minerals, which are the building blocks of our bodies. Fruits are high in vitamins but low in minerals. For this reason, vegetable juice is preferable when looking to rebuild one's body. Other important benefits to raw food are the live enzymes and quantity of antioxidants, which otherwise would be lost in the cooking process. Be aware as well that most of our diet should be consumed raw according to experts on our physiology. This is a lot to expect, of course; bear in mind that the majority of society has not been taught how to eat in this manner. However, raw vegetable jucing provides an avenue for consuming far greater amounts of raw food than an average person would ever eat in a day.

MICHELLE HONDA'S FAVORITE VEGETABLE JUICE FORMULA

4 pounds of carrots
1 apple

1 medium beet
Add dandelion, parsley or other comparable green

Do not peel the vegetables. Pare and trim any bad spots and/or tops and ends that are damaged. Do not mix fruit with vegetables; however, you are allowed an apple in a vegetable juice formula to increase the mixture's sweetness. This recipe makes enough for two adults. For one person, cut recipe in half and consume two cups.

Buy once a week (or as needed) and divide. One bunch of dandelion typically lasts 5 juice formulas. On occasion, add black radish and/or a portion of celery root. If these vegetables seem large, divide and reserve for another day or juicing time within the same day.

Drink 1 pint at a time *within an hour or less*. Makes 4 cups.

Vegetable juice is a quick and easy way to insert more raw food into your daily diet. You will become far less hungry and you may drink it often. It is fabulous as a weight loss companion. Your appetite center goes off after consuming this type of a liquid. Initially, drink only the quantity of juice that is tolerated by your bowels. If diarrhea is a problem, add adequate amounts of fiber such as ground flax seeds, psyllium husks or guar gum and lower consumption until the juice is tolerated. Please share with the whole family!

How to Take Michelle Honda's Vegetable Juice

Drink 1 pint a day (2 cups or 500 ml). Remember to drink it *as* you make it; do not store to drink later. It's best to take first thing in the morning for energy and nutritional support (although when diarrhea is presenting a great challenge, later in the day may be a better option). For a speedier healing process, drink this formula more than once a day. Powdered supplements may be added to this liquid, as well as any oils, or fiber like ground flax seeds, hemp powder, lactose-free whey powder or goat's whey. Shake and drink.

This drink is very healing and is restorative on a cellular level. You do not need to buy organic vegetables. If you wish to narrow it down to only one green, buy dandelion, and divide it up throughout several juice formulas. You may add additional greens like kale, if desired.

In the beginning, when diarrhea is a problem or bowel movements occur too frequently, add additional fiber, such as two tablespoons of ground flax seeds, to one or two cups (250–500 ml) of liquid. Fiber may need to be increased in between meals, while also accompanying a meal (in any liquid) when diarrhea is a constant problem, at least until the healing process takes hold. The goal of increasing fiber is to form a fecal mass, which in turn provides for less nutrient loss.

Initial Quick Start Program

To successfully treat a chronic condition, the individual who is suffering requires knowledge and guidance in order to promote a full understanding of why their body is reacting in the way that it is *and* how to remedy their aliment without medications.

Patients have become accustomed to taking prescription drugs. Adopting a new way of eating and treating symptoms naturally may be overwhelming in the beginning, mainly due to unfamiliar foods or remedies. Know that what I have presented within these pages works and works quickly. It all comes down to you—how much effort are you willing to put into a temporary change with long-lasting benefits? On initial query, I cannot recall getting anything less than an enthusiastic response of, "The quicker, the better!" Until the body starts to respond positively, some patients will have doubts whether healing medication-free is possible, since their only experience has been drugs (that lead to other drugs.)

What the Body Has Taught Me
The body has an amazing capacity to heal itself, so much so that I can hardly believe the results myself. I have come to learn just what is possible when the body as a whole is supported. When the body is enabled to do its job, even seemingly insurmountable feats of healing can be accomplished. I will have patients come in, prednisone and other drug prescriptions in hand to be filled, complaining of constant diarrhea and bleeding. And yet, they do not need to purchase the drugs. I also see many patients looking for options other than surgery. Once your symptoms subside and tissue is renewing, why would you need surgery? As a holistic doctor, my aim is always to help people who are drug-dependent become drug free. Your body does not function normally when on medication. For those who are already on several meds, a steady reduction takes place, coinciding with

the person's healing progress. This book alone should provide you with enough avenues, even some unrelated to gut dysbiosis, to assist you in reducing or eliminating many mainstream medications.

To Take the Fast Track or the Slow Road
The problem is a logical one. When you have a gut disease that disrupts the absorption of the food you *do* manage to eat, then limited dietary intake for a protracted period of time can further weaken the body. A common desire is for the body to be pain and symptom-free. The body cannot perform as fully or as quickly as you would like it to unless it is given back a lot of what it needs. The issue is that people are not taught how to feed their bodies adequately, making sure that it has the chance to perform optimally. Your body has much to teach you, rather than the other way round.

When desiring a speedier reversal of symptoms *and* a continuance of healing, consider the following: you *can* utilize less of my recommendations and heal at a slower pace. The choice is always yours. I have provided a protocol for the quickest disease reversal process I know, which involves treating all of your symptoms at once, as well as strengthening and supporting all the main body systems and functions. A tired, weak body cannot heal itself.

If you leave out crucial elements of my program, such as healing teas or herbs and vegetable juicing, your healing process will be significantly slower and more sporadic. If you feel compelled to avoid an aspect of my program, please make certain to substitute it with something else, to ensure that you get the missing nutrients. In this way, improvement will always be felt.

Ask yourself a few honest questions to help determine your comfort zone:

1. On a scale of 1 to 10, how badly do you want to get rid of the condition that plagues you?
2. How quickly do you want to heal?
3. Will you change your routine enough to accommodate the necessary different diet suggestions and healing remedies, to be taken at the appropriate times designated to provide the best results?

What Is Involved

1. A temporary change in routine, especially for the first month until symptoms have sufficiently subsided.

2. Following a new dietary plan that stops any further breakdown of the body by removing any food and beverage that either causes a worsening of symptoms or an over reactive immune response.

3. Keeping a food journal to determine what was taken into the body that caused an adverse reaction. The body usually reacts quickly, but delayed reactions do occur. Another reason for keeping a record of food intake is that, once you are eating a wider variety of food, you'll need to be sure that your balance of acid to alkaline foods is being considered to sustain optimum health. A diet of mostly starch and protein foods would indicate not nearly enough fruits and vegetables are being consumed.

4. Drinking raw vegetable juice, as this form of nutrition is necessary for a faster disease reversal. It provides the missing electrolytes, higher amounts of antioxidants, and easily absorbed vitamins and minerals. You are saving money by not having to purchase many of these nutrients, while also getting them in a far superior form which can be quickly utilized by the body. The more you juice, the faster you will heal. I do not suggest changing my formula until you are well healed. You may add extra greens but no additional fruit.

5. Healing teas or other naturally-sourced remedies.

6. Supplementation is normally required, especially for chronic conditions. These individuals have more food assimilation problems and more deficiencies. Dosages for some may need to be higher in the short term, followed by a few main ones which are necessary for all of us who live in industrialized locations where we do not grow our own food. Certain nutrients and fats are routinely missing in our diets.

If the body is not provided an adequate nutrition base, it cannot be expected to sustain us in a manner that we would all like. Throughout this book, you will learn what is required to maintain health and extended longevity.

What Initiates an Overeactive Immune Response Causing Diarrhea?
An example of something that can cause a repetitive autoimmune response is the body's reaction to the protein gluten, especially when it ends up where it should never be found. In the beginning, diarrhea or loose stools may be seen, which can quickly turn into a constant problem. A compromised intestinal tract is subject to many tiny unwanted substances that pass through its membranes into the blood. Immediately, the body recognizes these "intruders" and signals the immune system to jump into action. In such cases, the mantra of "once an intruder, always an intruder" seems to apply, and which can involve small proteins, along with other chemicals or allergens that venture where they do not belong. Gluten (and oftentimes dairy) are common culprits, and every time they show up, the immune system is on alert to protect the body by removing the "problem."

Gluten is not always the initial cause. Many people are gluten and dairy intolerant; however, for the majority of people that I routinely see something else precipitated the environment for which certain substances and foods are now deemed unfavorable. The most common causes are antibiotics, harsh or prolonged usage of medications, spinal or tail bone injury (this is especially the case with colitis) and psychological trauma, depression and stress. The gut reacts automatically to our emotions. Other offenders are bacteria, viruses, parasites and food poisoning.

Gluten Creates an Auto-Immune Disorder
Involving the Thyroid
There is another reason to pay attention to gluten, especially if you have determined that you are sensitive or intolerant to it. Gluten has an identical matrix to our thyroid tissue. The immune system is known to attack gluten and the thyroid gland simultaneously since it misreads it as being the same substance. This causes inflammation conditions in the thyroid gland, such as Hashimoto's disease and thyroiditis. The thyroid gland and adrenal glands are well documented in this book, as they play a paramount role in your healing and coping skills, as well as your future well-being.

Initial Quick Start Protocol for Acute or Chronic Symptoms: Crohn's,
Ulcerative Colitis (Pancolitis), Celiac, IBS and Diarrhea
The following segment is a condensed protocol to assist in quickly addressing many aspects of severe or very troublesome symptoms associated with gastrointestinal disorders. The following recommendations directly

address acute symptoms of diarrhea, inflammation, and bleeding, and look to boost the immune response, while correcting a few main nutrient deficiencies. The information below is described in more detail throughout this book.

All supplements are to be taken with food unless specified on the label. All minerals, such as zinc and magnesium, require a protein to be ingested at the time of consuming. (Refer to Chapter 10 for more information on magnesium.) Minerals require amino acids to carry and direct them on their designated path throughout the body. Since magnesium is the main element in the body performing many more functions than any other; it becomes crucial to further ensure the availability of this mineral by way of supplementation. The carrier protein for magnesium is frequently impaired with conditions like Crohn's disease and colitis, as well as other gut abnormalities. I have not noticed my dosage recommendations to be a problem in promoting diarrhea or loose stools. If you experience an adverse reaction, lower the dosage amounts and take more often.

Diarrhea and Bleeding
Argimony tincture is a very effective herbal remedy for diarrhea and bleeding. It even proves effective when symptoms are acute; all that is required is a higher initial dosage. For example, chronic diarrhea (with or without bleeding) may require 10 drops, four times over the first hour, followed by once hourly for 6–8 dosages, or every other hour over an 8 hour period. One teaspoon of argimony contains 60 drops. This is only a guide, which may be greatly increased or reduced in dosage. More drops may be taken at once if needed, for instance 25–30, and as often as needed. Once symptoms start to decline, the frequency of the dosage is lessened to maintain a level of continuance healing until it is no longer required. You should initially look for a reduction in the frequency of diarrhea or bowel movements and bleeding. Additional fiber will assist diarrhea. Refer to Chapter 11 for argimony product sources. Other herbs with astringent qualities include meadowsweet, bayberry, oak bark, and cranesbill. For more guidance, refer to the section of this chapter on fiber, and the sections in Chapter 13 detailing further choices in fiber.

Note that herbs do not work in the same way a medication would for the same symptom. They do not block as quickly as a drug; however, they do provide the same outcome over a period of time without the unwanted side effects incurred by drugs. Because drugs cannot grow tissue, complementary medicine along with nutrition enables the body to rebalance and restore itself. Drugs interrupt holistic pathways in the body, whereas whole natural sources do not.

Healing the Intestinal Lining

There are many herbal recommendations referenced in this book, suitable for most complaints associated with gastrointestinal problems and related conditions such as depression, anxiety, overuse of antibiotics, various forms of pain and inflammation and much more. Oftentimes, the job is accomplished with just a few remedies when the body as a whole is being addressed. The body is extremely proficient at healing itself when it is supported through nutrition, along with any extra supplemental nutrient requirements, and by not further breaking the body down. Originally, medicine came from a natural source; in this whole state, it can provide the necessary action to treat acute and chronic symptoms that plagues and prolongs an illness.

For healing intestinal tract tissues, I often recommend two herbs: comfrey root powder and slippery elm bark powder. Comfrey is known as the knitter of tissue. It greatly assists in healing up the holes in the gut and has many different properties and actions, including astringents for bleeding and diarrhea, as well as many others. Slippery elm is known for its soothing and demulcent properties. Comfrey and slippery elm may be combined together at once when making the recommended tea, as well as the amount needed for the day. The only draw back is that the tea mixture tends to become a bit gelatinous the longer it sits, mainly due to the slippery elm powder.

Herbs such as these (or others with the same effects) enhance the healing process, which in turn reduces acute and chronic symptoms by allowing the body to remain balanced and normalized in its healing process.

Once a healing process commences, the symptoms should reduce as the patient becomes much stronger and hopeful. By adhering to a diet protocol until the gut is fully healed, a full reversal is attained. Long before this stage, the need for traditional medicine falls by the wayside.

Comfrey root decoction tea: 1 teaspoon per cup, and drink 3 cups throughout the day. Bring to a boil, and simmer for 15–20 minutes. Purchase the leaf if you cannot find the root (though the root is stronger in its healing properties). Refer to Chapter 11 for comfrey and herb sources.

Slippery elm decoction tea: 1 teaspoon per cup and drink 3 times a day. Bring to a boil and simmer for 15 minutes. Slippery elm bark is easily accessed in most supplement stores.

Combination Tea: Combine ½ teaspoon of each herb (comfrey root and slippery elm bark) per cup of water and prepare accordingly.

Retention Enema: In cases of colitis involving the sigmoid colon region, apply the same formula in a retention enema for speedier, direct healing. Refer to Chapter 11 for directions on how to perform this process.

Supplementation
Initial supplementation is often necessary for addressing deficiencies and malnourishment, as well as to promote a speedier recovery:

Nutritional Flaked Yeast: 1 tablespoon, twice a day (or if taking Tortula, a similar type of supplement, take 1 teaspoon twice a day). Nutritional flaked yeast is a complete protein source and has all B vitamins. Buy in bulk or in a container if you prefer (most health food stores sell it in a bulk form). Kosher varieties are also available. Add to any liquid or sprinkle on food. For health maintenance, continue some form of B vitamin supplement.

L-Tyrosine (Thyroid support): Choose a reputable brand. Take one 500 mg capsule three times a day for one month then reduce to one capsule twice a day (unless your energy has not sufficiently returned). Continue taking one a day for health maintenance. Note that this is not recommended for conditions of hyperthyroidism or Hashimoto's disease.

Liquid Iodine Drops (Thyroid support): Use as directed by your product of choice. It can also be combined with other minerals, or taken in the form of liquid kelp. Not recommended for conditions of hyperthyroidism or Hashimoto's disease until the gland/body has completely normalized. A blood test will help determine the stage of recovery.

Endocrine support: Multi-glandular desiccated gland extracts. Take two capsules twice times a day or as directed by the manufacturer. For future health maintenance, a supplement such as this will provide good organ and gland support. A dosage of half the normal recommendation taken five days a week is a helpful option for promoting ongoing health.

Zinc: One 25 mg tablet taken twice a day for 3–4 weeks, and then reduce to one a day. With an onset of illness, increase zinc; otherwise, taking once a day is endorsed for maintaining health.

Magnesium citrate: 300 mg, taken three times a day. This dosage may be increased or decreased, depending on the severity of your gut dysbiosis. Other forms of magnesium may be taken if its absorbability is enhanced. A low dosage of magnesium is highly suggested for future health maintenance.

Colostrum: 2 capsules taken twice a day will boost immunity and enhance tissue repair. It also helps to heal holes in the intestinal tract. Reduce or stop when healing is well on its way.

L-Glutamine: One 500 mg capsule taken 2–3 times a day provides for rapid intestinal cell replication. Reduce to one capsule a day when all gut symptoms have stabilized or until symptoms no longer occur.

Fish oil: Take two 500–600 mg capsules three times a day for one month, and then reduce to two capsules taken twice a day as healing improves. Increase dosage for pain and inflammation as needed. If taken as a liquid, take 1 teaspoon (if the dosage is 1000 mg per teaspoon). Apply accordingly. Refer to Chapter 10 to read more about its role in healing and maintenance of health.

Flax seed oil: 1 tablespoon twice a day, taken in liquid or on food (such as a salad, in place of olive oil). Do not heat essential oils.

Probiotics: Two capsules taken twice a day or as directed by your brand of choice (dairy-free is available). Always incorporate some form of probiotic into your diet on an ongoing basis. Once fully healed, this does not need to be consumed daily. A normal recommended dosage may be taken 3–5 days a week and omitted for short periods of time (as when on a holiday).

Liquid Chlorophyll: 2 teaspoons three times a day in water. Sip throughout the day. Provides minerals and alkalization, and is great for all acid conditions and anemia. For anemic conditions that are ferritin-related (iron) chlorophyll is wonderful and does not cause constipation.

B-12: Take 1200 mcg a day (for Crohn's disease and colitis patients) or as directed by your doctor. Some individuals require regular shots of B-12, which will be performed by their physician.

Coconut oil: This is optional, but taking 1 teaspoon per day can provide health benefits. This oil may be heated and used for cooking.

Observe the Results
As you initiate the new program, observe and monitor any changes in your fecal matter over the first few days (up to one week). In the beginning, you should be looking for any improvement, which includes increased energy and a reduction in diarrhea, bleeding, and the frequency of bowel movements and pain. If diarrhea remains too persistent, the diet must be more carefully monitored. It may also simply be a case of severe inflammation, which can account for pain, gas and bloating from just about anything being consumed in the early stages of healing. The current status of the intestinal tract is a factor, as well as specific foods or substance triggers.

Unfortunately, there can be many factors that may slow down your initial success in the first week or two. These may include how depleted and low functioning your body has become. In such cases, continue with the more restricted dietary recommendations and only begin reintroducing food items (one at a time) if you feel sure that they are not a major intolerance. Supplementation is required to restore your systems, especially if your food intake has been very limited up until now.

Prepare Food for Easy Digestion
Until sufficient improvement has occurred, meals must be prepared for easy digestibility. Nourishing soups, raw food juices, protein smoothies and stews that are coarsely blended are all great options. Acidic foods like tomato sauce, processed fruit juices or large quantities of animal protein should be avoided. Herbal teas, especially those listed in this book, are welcomed.

Herbs may be required (such as passion flower or chamomile) in the form of a tea or liquid tincture if your stomach is spastic, or vomiting is occurring. Other choices for anti-spasmodic action include hops, lobelia, mistletoe, skullcap and valerian. Remedies such as these and more are referenced in this book. Refer to Chapter 11 for product sources.

Anxiety
Conditions of anxiety or stress can automatically trigger bowel movements—as many with IBS can attest. Refer to the Chapter 8 for more guidance.

Initial Food Restrictions

Omit the following: gluten; dairy without probiotics; sugar; corn and all corn products; coffee; alcohol; wine; processed food; junk food; large amounts of any animal protein at one meal; soda; nuts and seeds (unless ground or in a butter form); and any food item or substance that you are already aware of as being a problem. For a guide, refer to the diet section for foods to consume and avoid. If you are absolutely sure that you can tolerate certain foods listed as permitted, you can include them in your diet (with the exception of gluten, at least initially).

Initial Recommended Reading in *Reverse Gut Diseases Naturally*

You should seek to read as much of the book as possible while incorporating the initial protocol to provide for an understanding of the imbalances taking place within your gut and body. For quick reference, refer to the following:

- For healing the intestinal tract and minimizing symptoms, follow the diet recommendations in Chapter 12.

- For information about leaky gut syndrome, refer to Chapter 4.

- Initial Protocol: When reading Chapter 5, read the whole chapter—not just the quick start to the initial protocol.

- For information on juicing raw foods and the benefits of carrot juice, refer to Chapters 5 and 9.

- To become familiar with the different types of fiber and other plant components that are fiber related, refer to Chapters 12 and 13. Look for guar gum, pectin and locust bean (for more than one choice) particularly when the gut is highly inflamed or sensitive, and coupled with diarrhea.

- For information referring to diarrhea and bleeding, familiarize yourself with the protocol for diarrhea and associated remedies as well as how to make various herbal teas provided in Chapter 11.

- For information relating to the thyroid and adrenal glands, including the problems involved in testing the thyroid, and how to take care of this area of your endocrine system, refer to Chapter 2.

- For information relating to omega 3 fatty acid's role in healing, health and longevity, refer to Chapter 10.

- For information relating to colostrum, including the ways in which colostrum boosts the immune system and tissue repair, refer to Chapter 9.
- To familiarize with what replaces antibiotics, pain and inflammation medications, including the herbs that heal and constrict for diarrhea and bleeding, as well as those for stress, anxiety/depression, etc., refer to Chapters 7, 8 and 11.

Plant Fiber

About Fiber

The term "fiber" is a bit of a misnomer, since many sources of fiber are not, in reality, fibrous. Upon taking a closer look at the constituents found in plants, fiber takes on many characteristics beyond the typical description of soluble or insoluble fiber. Fiber's role is being hailed as the nutrients we take into our body, and is being widely used to assist in healing and regulating functions and systems throughout the whole body.

Not all fiber suits all needs, and certain health conditions demand a particular type of fiber to provide a desired result. Fiber must be compatible with the body in order to provide the desired benefit without promoting unwanted symptoms.

Through patient and public interactions, I notice a great deal of misconception surrounding fiber. People are unsure as to whether they should take it or not, even though many times it would assist in restoring their body's balance. And yet, people are preconditioned towards thinking fiber is only for the benefit of constipation, and that it will surely cause the reverse condition if taken.

As will be demonstrated throughout this book, fiber promotes stabilization for many substances taken into the body, along with providing nutrition while improving the healing and health status of several conditions.

Nutritional Benefit of Edible Fiber

Too often, fiber is thought to be nutrient poor. Various sources of fiber fall into different groups, providing a wide variety of uses. It is nice to know that some plants can provide the necessary health benefits while still offering an abundance of nutrition. There are many misconceptions surrounding the topic of fiber, and what it does or does not do for a particular problem. One such area of concern—where there should be none—is about the blocking of vitamin and mineral absorption. Plant fiber does not restrict the absorption of vitamins and minerals; in fact, the evidence seems to suggest otherwise!

Fermentable Fiber
A category of fiber, referred to as fermentable, has unique qualities as compared to other types of fiber. The highest fermentable fibers are groups of polysaccharides such as beta-glucans, pectin, natural gums, oligosaccharides (a group of short chained or simple sugars), inulin and others. These fermentable sources improve the absorption of minerals, in particular calcium, which is great news for anyone suffering with osteoporosis.

Phytates in plants have been found to reduce the absorption of some minerals and vitamins (which is not to be confused with fiber content). A few examples include calcium, zinc, magnesium and vitamin C.

Fiber Contains Beta-Glucans
Beta-glucan is a highly prized nutrient among the health conscious public. The following examples are sources of soluble fiber with the benefit of beta-glucans.

- Whole grain barley
- Dry milled barley
- Oat bran
- Rolled oats
- Oatrim
- Whole oat flour
- Psyllium husks (purity no less than 95 percent)

> Refer to Chapter 13 for information on gluten-free fiber.

How Does Fiber Help Diarrhea?
Hopefully, you are starting to notice that fiber wears many hats, yet they all fall under the umbrella of fiber. All these varying types of fiber offer individual benefits, from nutrition to assisting with balancing a wide variety of ailments. The first condition discussed in regards to fiber usage will be overly frequent bowl movements verging on chronic diarrhea. Initially,

fiber is as important as any constricting agent. There are a host of problems surrounding diarrhea, which stem from nutrients and electrolytes leeching out of the body, up to and including the discomfort of inflammation, gas, bloating and ocassionally even bleeding.

Diarrhea and Malnourishment

The first concern in regards to diarrhea is malnourishment. The body cannot fight back or remain strong when the food being eaten is passing through the intestinal tract without adequate time allowed for absorption. The immune response is overreactive and quickly becomes overworked. Typically, the dietary intake for anyone with diarrhea is very limited. The longer the problem persists, the more irritated the stomach and intestinal lining become, to the point where it becomes very hard to find something to eat that does not cause symptoms of discomfort. The more deficient the diet becomes, the more exhausted the immune system becomes.

Envision the immune system coping with many antigens like gluten, lactose, chemicals and drugs that are even now slipping through the permeable intestinal tract into areas they are never meant to be found in. This scenario creates an immune response which now lists these antigens as undesired items in preparation for when they show up again. You now not only have to deal with diarrhea but the problem of substances and diet that will continue to cause the body to eliminate items that were once tolerated but are currently being viewed as a problem.

How to Implement Fiber

Fiber is necessary to reduce the flow of body fluids and promote the absorption of tolerated food and the extra supplementation being taken to help rebalance the body and strengthen it. The first step is to remove any and all items that have been shown to be a problem. Vegetable and green juices and smoothies are very helpful in lightening the load on the digestive process and provide an avenue for easily digestible nutrition where whole food supplements and other nutrients can be added.

To ensure bowel tolerance of liquids or food, adjustments may be required in the amount and frequency of fiber being taken. Also, the type of fiber may need to be changed if it seems to be bothersome. For instance, ground flax seeds have enormous nutritional benefit, yet occasionally a really sensitive stomach or gut will repel almost everything. But giving up is not an option; in such cases, temporally switch to a gelatinous-type fiber like guar gum, pectin and locust bean. Refer to Chapter 13 for information on fiber such as these and similar ones, including memicellulose and vegetable gums.

Recommendations on what should accompany fiber, namely naturally astringent plants and their properties, will be covered under the topics of diarrhea and bleeding. Regardless of how well a remedy may work, fiber should be integrated into the program.

Example for Diarrhea and How Often to Consume Fiber
The worse the condition and frequency of diarrhea is, the more often fiber ought to be consumed. Add fiber to liquid, divided up throughout the day. If someone is having 10–20 visits to the bathroom in a day then the frequency of fiber intake should be experimented with over the first two days, up to a week.

> Before I continue on, realize that a debilitated person will respond more slowly to this program, until the level of nutrition is consistent enough to stabilize the symptoms and boost the immune system (and the body as a whole). As the body becomes better able to retain nourishment, it will become stronger and more energized. A tired body cannot heal itself. The fiber serves as a medium to assist the body in slowing down the excess fluid being flushed into the intestinal tract to remove unwanted substances.
>
> The results will be very favorable if all intolerances have been removed. The first couple of days can still be bumpy depending on the degree of inflammation, but in such cases high-quality, easily digestible nutrition is paramount to enhance tissue renewal. Try to be patient; the body's capacity to heal itself is nothing short of remarkable—when sufficiently supported.

Adding Fiber to Liquid and Puréed Foods
To reiterate, the protocol described in this chapter is for frequent bowel movements and chronic diarrhea. For milder conditions, simply reduce the frequency of fiber intake throughout the day. Start by juicing vegetables or other well tolerated liquids and add other items when appropriate (such as a supplement or omega 3 fatty acid) along with the fiber. In the morning, start with 2 tablespoons of finely ground flax seeds (or other gentle fiber of choice) to one or two glasses of liquid, juice or broth. Yogurt is great (if tolerated) for setting up the stomach in the presence of severe

nausea or inflammation. It may also be added to your liquids or non-heated liquid food items (such as soups or smoothies). Liquid chlorophyll in water is another good choice.

Repeat every two hours. Take between meals, or else just before or after you eat or consume food until a stool starts to form. This will take a day or two (unless diarrhea is still persistent). The goal is to take in enough fiber to firm up the feces and to reduce the number of bowel movements in a day. Also, consider the quantity of juice consumed at any given time. Drinking slowly may be required, along with limiting one's self to smaller amounts at a given time. Reduce fiber frequency according to how your fecal matter appears and how often elimination is required. Sometimes, constipation may appear to be a gift. If the fecal matter becomes too firm, cut back on the number of times fiber is taken throughout the day. It is best at meal time (if constipation is present) or less frequently (if the diarrhea is under control).

Vegetable juice and similar liquids are a food source to the body which doesn't require all the usual work of digestion. Many times, people do not realize that liquid food is still food, and not just water to be eliminated by the kidneys. However, it will still stimulate peristalsis in the bowel. When food is being eaten, it triggers a natural process which secretes digestive enzymes and moves food along.

Other Health Benefits of Fiber
The applications of fiber involve numerous physiological processes, including inflammation, which promote health and wellness:

- Soluble fiber produces short chain fatty acids, which are involved in the regulation of glucose, through the process of fermentation. This fermented fiber provides nourishment to colonocytes and serves as a protective barrier to the intestinal mucosal layer, inhibiting inflammation. They are also expressed in the production of antibodies, leukocytes, cytokines and the lymph system, thus playing a key role in immune protection. Short chain fatty acids are butyrate, propionate, and acetate. Their actions upon the body are as followed:
    - Butyrate is the major energy source for colonocytes.
    - Propionate is designed for utilization by the liver.

- Acetate penetrates the peripheral circulation to be transformed by peripheral tissues.
- Soluble and insoluble fiber improves several aspects of gastrointestinal health:
  - Fermented soluble fiber has a positive impact on colonic microflora.
  - Relieves constipation by increasing fecal mass and improves transit time in the large colon.
  - Slows down carbohydrate and sugar absorption, improving glucose tolerance (GTF) and insulin response.
- Soluble fiber stabilizes blood glucose levels by affecting insulin release and liver regulation of glycogen breakdown.
- Soluble fiber reduces LDL cholesterol levels and associated risk factors of coronary heart disease.
- Fiber lowers hypertension/blood pressure
- Fiber lowers the incidence of certain cancers; in particular, colon cancer.
- Fiber benefits weight loss in several ways:
  - Slows down sugar absorption.
  - Binds to fat, preventing its reasborption back through the intestines.
  - Increases the sensation of satiety, feeling full longer.

Raw Food is Nature's Way to Better Gut Health

The evolution of our diet and the way we prepare our food is alarmingly opposed to our genetic makeup. Our inherent nature is to be predominately alkaline. We achieve this by eating a diet in accordance to our body's natural laws; in other words, our diet should consist of 80 percent fruits and vegetables, of which about 70 percent should be raw, according to experts. The quality and longevity of our life depends on meeting our body's nutritional needs on a regular basis.

We will explore the reasoning behind the above statement, including the benefits seen when this dietary regime is applied correctly. We will also examine the consequences of *not* implementing such a plan. Finally, we'll be taking a look at the benefits of raw juice, while touching briefly on embracing a total raw food diet.

Our Body's Physiology in Relation to Digestion
Let's start by taking a brief look at our physiology. By simply observing our digestive process, the way in which we chew food and the purpose of our long digestive tract is patterned for the slow breakdown and absorption of plant material. This is, by design, set up for a predominately alkaline diet consisting of mostly fruits and vegetables. Our body requires food with its life force still intact in order for regeneration to take place, and the functioning of our systems depends on many of the elements which are forever lost during the cooking process.

What is a Raw Food Diet?
The raw food diet is based on whole, unprocessed and uncooked fresh foods. A typical food list includes fruit, vegetables, sprouts, seeds, nuts, beans, dried fruit, coconut milk and seaweed. The percentage of raw food required to be considered a raw diet isn't far off the normal healthy eating regime: generally 75 percent of one's diet must be living or raw (although there are individuals whose lifestyle involves 100 percent raw food intake).

Health Benefits of Raw and Alkaline Foods
Osteoporosis is directly linked to the acid/alkaline balance of the body. When we eat an acidic food, such as protein, it causes our system to become more acidic. The parathyroid gland (which regulates the body's acid/alkaline balance) in turn robs our bones and tissues of calcium to bring the blood back to its healthy alkaline state. This gland is granted full control over our body's infrastructure, so much so that it can impact our skeletal system, promoting bone loss in an effort to maintain an inherent balance. There are additional issues involving osteoporosis; however, diet must be addressed to prevent bone loss and to maintain proper pH levels.

Digestive problems are common as we age, primarily due to reduced enzyme activity from the age of forty. However, in recent years increased instances of digestive problems are mostly due to our body's digestive enzymes not having been supported with living plant enzymes. Incorporating raw food into each meal supports the digestive process, while cooking food above 116°F destroys the enzymes in food that can assist in the digestive process and the absorption of food. The nutritional value is also greatly diminished.

Raw foods rejuvenate, cleanse, raise oxygen blood levels and energize our bodies. The aging process is slowed immensely and vitality is felt throughout your whole being. The body becomes light; bowel cleansing is enhanced; circulation is increased; mental clarity improves; and a zest for life is renewed. Weight loss is virtually guaranteed, as is beautiful skin and reduced risk of heart disease and cancer. Other concerns in the area of diabetes and high cholesterol/triglyceride levels are all benefited by a raw food diet.

Nutritional Benefits of Raw Food and Sprouts
Raw food and sprouts are very nutritious and offer great health benefits by providing us with a wide spectrum of color, encompassing a wide variety of phytochemicals and nutrients. Other benefits include fiber, enzymes, antioxidants, proteins, nitrosamines, bioflavonoids, vitamins, minerals and low trans-fat and saturated fat.

Sprouts are living foods that have concentrated amounts of phytochemicals and antioxidants, which can protect us from disease and slow the aging process. For example, the saponins found in alfalfa have been shown to lower bad cholesterol. Researchers at John Hopkins University School of Medicine have discovered that broccoli sprouts contain high amounts of a natural cancer fighting compound.

Juicing Raw Foods for Cleansing and Restoring Health
Juicing may well be a cutting edge therapy for reclaiming and maintaining our health. Drinking raw juices is a fast way for the body to obtain vitamins and minerals, and an easy way to boost your daily intake of raw food.

Cleansing and detoxifying are hot topics in today's media. But the best form of cleansing is through whole, unadulterated vegetable and fruit juices. This form of nutrition is already metabolically broken down by the fine root fibers for easy assimilation. Juicing is highly recommended for various cleansing programs because of its condensed nutritional value and live enzymatic activity.

One example is a lymph system cleanse, which is of particular importance since, along with our liver, the lymph system is one of our body's primary detoxification systems. Our lymph is often overloaded with toxic material from air pollution, food additives and poisonous sprays. In order to clean the lymph stream, specific minerals must be available. Fortunately, minerals and other beneficial nutrients such as phytochemicals are abundantly available in vegetable and fruit juices.

Raw juices (especially a vegetable formula) are wonderful for raising the immune system. An immune-boosting juice formula would include above ground and below ground plants such as carrots as the main ingredient, with beets, dandelions, or parsley, and even black radish, celery root or potato added occasionally. These foods are extremely valuable to your liver, kidney, immune system, blood and connective tissue. Typically, fruits are not mixed with vegetables; however, as has been stated, the inclusion of one apple in the formula listed in this chapter is permissible (for added flavor). Remember, all juices should be consumed within one hour of being made.

A breakfast fruit juice formula with protein may include the following:

> 2 cups freshly made fruit juice of choice (such as apple,
>   pineapple or berries)
>
> 1 tablespoon of your favorite nut or seed butter
>
> ½ cup fresh fruit
>
> 1 tablespoon flax seed oil
>
> 1 raw egg yolk or ½ cup of plain yogurt (optional).

If desired, sweeten with raw honey to taste.

Cooking Methods of Raw Food

Cooking and preparation techniques enhance the variety and digestibility of an uncooked diet. Usually, the following methods are employed: sprouting seeds, grains and beans; juicing fruits and vegetables; soaking nuts; reconstituting dried fruits; and blending and dehydrating food.

There is a misconception regarding the length of preparation time when introducing either a raw food diet or incorporating more of the same. The fact is that in many instances, less time is required to prepare a delicious, nutritionally balanced meal using raw food. The substitution of foods palatable for non-cooking is the biggest hurdle.

Some common areas of adjustment are as follows:
- Spaghetti is often replaced with spaghetti squash, thinly sliced zucchini, sprouted nut seeds such as almonds or shredded carrots.
- Spaghetti sauce may be pesto (raw basil and olive oil), or crushed tomatoes, raw herbs, garlic and olive oil.

- Fats are usually replaced with cold pressed oils, coconut butter and avocado.
- Better cheese choices are from goat's cheese or cheese made from nuts and seeds. Hummus with raw vegetables is a healthy snack.
- Replacing starch wraps with a lettuce leaf are wonderful for lunch and benefits the waist line. Take a lettuce leaf, fill it with your favorite vegetables (try to include sprouts), spread on tahini, and a small amount of your favorite dressing.

Particular attention should be paid to ensure adequate levels of B12 and protein when consuming a raw food diet. Raw food, juicing and sprouts will help anyone reach their highest level of health and well-being. Any initiative made to include more raw food into your daily intake is a measure taken towards better health. Juicing provides obvious benefits for sensitive and inflamed intestinal tracts. It also addresses the problem of malnourishment.

CHAPTER SIX

Complete Case Histories for Guidance Through the Healing Process

NTEGRATING CASE HISTORIES this early into a book is not common practice. Nevertheless, I have several reasons for wanting to share this information with you at this time. One reason is that the majority of this information has applications for several similar symptom complaints. There are also special cases, when a gut problem is *not* labeled as a rare type of condition, but for which (due to extended reasons of impaired healing) the following restricted dietary plan would be very helpful. In such cases, the restricted diet would only need to be applied long enough to ensure an initial healing process.

You will find two very comprensive case histories in this chapter, which have similar, yet slightly different disease complaints. Included with each is a step-by–step overview of their healing processes as well as all dietary and healing remedies.

The first case history spanned over several months while the second case history healed in a matter of weeks. You will notice major differences in their complaints as well as the length of time they have had to endure them. You will also notice a vastly different healing protocol that has evolved since the time of the first case history. Regardless of symptom complaints, the main consideration between these two examples is the second Crohn's/fistula patient's program. By predominantly using the Quick Start Program coupled with diet intervention, the healing process was rapidly reduced and the patient is now living medication-free. As with both cases, you will view all the stages of their healing progress that encompasses all aspects of my recommendations in their therapy.

Be aware that the first case history's protocol does not fall into the category of an average dietary program for inflammatory bowel disease (although it may initially have application for many Crohn's and colitis patients). The subsequent information will be quite comprehensive, and should be viewed as an example of a severe case of Crohn's Type 'A' condition. Any of the following recommendations *may* be used by individuals with similar symptoms such as pain, abscesses, fistulas, diarrhea, gas or bloating. A diet for all other type of gut disorders, including inflammatory bowel diseases, would not be as restrictive. Their diets may include grain replacements or whole grain gluten-free products.

Supplementation varies from one disorder to another. The quantity and amount of supplements taken in the following case history could very well be different for another, similar condition. Supplements in all forms as recommended in this book may be combined with one another or taken singularly, with a variance in dosage.

Sometimes, when encountering acute and prolonged symptoms that have not been responding to foods and items that are deemed safe, a short-term elimination diet such as this one may be beneficial, until a decrease in symptoms occurs. The diet in this case history is an example of a more uncommon condition where the patient's eating plan will always be very limited, as compared to most people who suffer with Crohn's disease and Ulcerative colitis. The dietary regime that a Type 'A' Crohn's person must follow is far more restricted than any other gut disorders that I have ever dealt with and requires strict adherence on the part of the patient.

CASE HISTORY: Type 'A' Crohn's Disease (2006)

I would like to preface this by saying that the number of appointments within this case history is far from normal. The average number of appointments (prior to reading this book) in treating these types of ailments is two to four appointments. With the availability of the information retained in this book, the appointment pattern should hopefully be reduced to one to three visits.

The case history displayed below is one of the few exceptions that did not follow the normal appointment protocol, partly due to the patient's desire to see me on a regular basis, as well as other complications requiring attention. Take note of the patient's vast improvement as it occurred over five appointments. After the fifth appointment, the main focus of her treatment plan centered on renal abscesses and fistulas, all of which had been a long standing problem. Since the time frame of this case history, my work with gastrointestinal complaints has greatly expanded, which has lead to my consistently redefining my program to promote a quicker disease reversal for my patients and a lighter protocol.

A female patient in her mid forties came to me, presenting with a long history of Crohn's disease. Her complaints included much discomfort from anal fistulas and an abscess, mild bleeding, gas, low libido, no energy, diarrhea and difficulty finding food that didn't trigger symptoms of gas, pain, diarrhea or indigestion. She had been treated by gastroenterologists for years, with little progress. Upon answering my questions, I determined that the woman had type 'A' Crohn's disease, which describes someone with a strong inherited weakness (see Chapter 4 for more information on Type 'A' Chron's disease). This patient had been taking medications for this disorder for years, and her current medicine profile included commonly prescribed drugs for the condition in the form of anti-inflammatories and antibiotics. (Refer to the patient's case history questionnaire for a list of her medications and foods that she had been eating).

My goal with every patient is to raise their level of health to the point where medication is no longer necessary, while managing the ailment or imbalance within their individual parameters.

First Appointment

Patient's Health History
The following is a question and answer dialog between the patient and Dr. Honda.

Q: How long have you had these symptoms?
A: 20 years.

Q: How many oxygen treatments, if any?
A: 20 hours; each session went 1 to 2 hours.

Q: What degree of success?
A: Fistula reduced by 15 percent, and not as painful.

Q: Did your mother have measles during her pregnancy with you?
A: No.

Q: Have you had surgery?
A: Yes; a rubber ring slipped through fistulas involving surgery to form a
    new opening for the ring to be put in. *(This occurred more than once in
    her health history).*

Q: Where is your inflammation located?
A: Intestines, especially the lower anal area due to diarrhea, fistulas and
    abscess.

Q: What supplements are you taking?
A: None currently.

Q: Do you have a sweet tooth?
A: Yes.

Q: How severe is your gas, bloating, diarrhea or abdominal pain?
A: No pain. Diarrhea is a problem—5–6 times a day.

Q: What foods cause gas, bloating, diarrhea, or abdominal pain?
A: Carbohydrates and fiber.

Q: How many servings of starches and sugars do you eat in a day? What
    are they?
A: Bread, two white slices with peanut butter and jam. Decaf coffee with
    half and half cream. Lunch of two slices of white bread with cold cuts.
    Water to drink. Dinner of wheat pasta, and bread 2–3 slices. Sweets,
    chocolate and cake.

Q: How many vegetables? What are they?
A: Virtually no vegetables. Afraid of diarrhea. Asparagus is ok.

Q: Fruits—how many? What are they?
A: Afraid to try bananas, due to problems in the past. Strawberries, grapes
    and melons.

Q: Proteins—how many? What are they?
A: Peanut butter, eggs, cold cuts; all meats and fish.

Q: Dairy consumption?
A: Not a problem. I do not eat yogurt.

Q: Drinks?
A: Decaf coffee, no alcohol, soda once a week or less. No fruit juice.

Q: Junk foods?
A: Candy, chips and garlic are ok—no popcorn, no nuts and no spicy foods. Hot pepper in any form is a problem.

Q: Did you have recurrent antibiotic pneumonia that was preceded by the Crohn's in every case? *(Antibiotics, as many know, increase fungal infection. Most antibiotics are mycotoxins-fungal derivatives).*
A: No.

Q: Mycotoxins are found in our grain food, especially corn. Do you eat corn products? *(Anyone who has consumed antibiotics, grains or sugars has a comprised immune system with this type of gut disorder).*
A: No.

Q: Do you take antibiotics?
A: Yes.

Q: Have you gone through severe emotional stress?
A: No.

Q: Did your symptoms exist before the stress?
A: Does not apply.

Q: Do you have leaky gut?
A: Unknown. *(I determined the answer was yes).*

Q: Do you have any allergies? Name them.
A: Unknown.

Q: Do you smoke?
A: No.

Medication
Q: Are you taking any of the following?
Q: Sulfasalazine. *(This is the most common).*
A: Yes.

Q: Mesalamine; if one cannot tolerate sulfasalazine, you may be put on mesalamine drugs, generally known as S-ASA agents.

A: Yes.

Q: Corticosteroids for inflammation, but which can cause serious side effects, including greater susceptibility to infection.

A: Currently no.

Q: 6-mercaptopurine and a related drug azathioprine are immune-suppressing drugs. They work by blocking the immune reaction that contributes to inflammation. Side effects include nausea, vomiting, diarrhea and a person's resistance to infection is lowered.

A: No.

Q: Remicade, for the treatment of moderate to severe Crohn's that do not respond to mesalamine substances, corticosteroids, immunosuppressive drugs and for the treatment of open, draining fistulas.

A: Not currently. (*The patient had been prescribed Remicade. Holding off on taking the drug to see how successful Michelle Honda's program turns out.*)

Q: Infliximab is an anti-tumors or necrosis factor (TNF) substance. TNF is a protein produced by the immune system which may cause inflammation associated with Crohn's. Anti-TNF removes the TNF from the bloodstream before it reaches the intestines, thereby preventing inflammation. Safety and efficacy of long-term use is not established.

A: No.

Q: Antibiotics, which treat bacterial infection.

A: Yes.

Q: Budersonide, a new corticosteroid that appears to be as effective as other corticosteroids, but causes fewer side effects.

A: No.

Q: Methotexate and cyclosporine—immunosuppressive drugs that may be useful; they appear to work faster than traditional immunosuppressive drugs.

A: No.

Q: Natalizumab is an experimental drug that decreases inflammation by binding to immune cells and preventing them from leaving the bloodstream and reaching the areas of inflammation.

A: No.

The patient is taking the following medications:

Antibiotic: Cipro, 500 mg, twice a day

Flagyl: 500 mg, twice a day

Pentasa: Two 500 mg doses, four times a day

Uenatetrenone: One dose, twice a day

Patient's Daily Regime

The Initial Protocol is included in the patient's therapy. Note that this is *not* the quick start program, as treatment protocols continued to evolve. The patient was instructed to select foods only from those listed under "Dietary Suggestions for Crohn's Disease, Ulcerative Colitis and Celiac Disease."

The following recommendations are designed to incorporate further additions as the healing process dictates, and the initial recommendations may be either increased or decreased. The program will include a diet to be determined upon the tolerance and symptoms of the patient. Also, the patient's complaints and discomforts will be addressed.

Note: Other types of inflammatory bowel disorder and other gut complaints such as irritable bowel syndrome may and often do have much more leeway with food allowances. Check the patient's sixth appointment for a sample of the patient's current daily eating regime up until that appointment.

Continuing First Appointment
When reviewing this patient's health history questionnaire, I noticed the high amount of carbohydrates and little to no vegetables and fruit. The following diet is designed to address the imbalances in this diet.

Diet
- Michelle Honda's vegetable juice formula: 1 quart per day; 1 pint in the morning and 1 pint in the afternoon or at lunch
- ½ cup plain yogurt (in the morning)
- Lunch and dinner to include protein along with well-cooked, tolerated vegetables or homemade soup

- Colostrum: 1 capsule, three times a day (must be a quality product)
- Multi-glandular desiccated extract: 1 capsule, twice a day
- Proteolytic enzyme therapy: 5 capsules, three times a day (taken on an empty stomach)
- Zinc: One 30 mg capsule, twice a day
- Kelp: 1 tablet a day
- Vitamin C: One 500 mg capsule, three times a day
- Acidophilus and bifidus: 2 capsules, twice a day
- Fish oil: One 600 mg gel capsule, three times a day
- Whey powder: 2 scoops, three times a day
- Salad dressing: apple cider vinegar and oil
- Ginger tea: 3 cups per day

Medications
- Cipro: 1 dose, twice a day
- Flagyl: 1 dose twice a day
- Pentasa: 2 pills, 2–4 times a day
- Sitz bath: for abscess and fistula; made with flaxseeds and witch hazel
    - Boil 3 tablespoons of flax seeds in 3 cups of water. Simmer for 10 minutes and strain. Sitz bath, flaxseed tea with a few drops of witch hazel

Patient is also visiting a health food store for carbohydrate-free snacks or other food items, as well as whey powder that is lactose-free.

Second Appointment (2 weeks later)
Changes and additions/ patient's progress and questions:

Progress: Patient's energy is up considerably. Symptoms are all minimizing. The patient is very encouraged. Patient decreased drug intake on her own accord.

Drug reduction: Patient reduced her Pentasa from eight pills a day down to six pills a day.

Supplement profile is the same with a few changes and additions below.

- Vegetable juice: 1 cup, three times a day
- Aloe vera gel: 2 tablespoons added to juice when consumed
- Ginger and yarrow tea: 3 cups throughout the day
- White willow bark: 240 mg as needed for pain or inflammation
- Boswellia: 350 mg, three times a day
- Anti-viral formula herbal tincture: 10 ml twice a day on the tongue or in liquid form for 2 weeks
- Stopped antibiotics

Third Appointment (4 weeks later)
Changes and additions/patient's progress and questions:

Progress: The patient continues to feel much better.

Drug: Pentasa reduced to five pills per day. Patient was able to discontinue the antibiotics. I replaced them with an anti-viral natural supplement formula.

Previous appointment protocol (other than the following changes) continues unchanged.
- Reducing anti-viral formula format (first week, 25 ml twice a day; second week reduced to once a day)
- SAM-e: 1–2 capsules a day, or as needed
- Liquid chlorophyll: 2 teaspoons in water sipped throughout the day (1–3 glasses)
- Zinc: reduced to once a day
- Fish oil: increased to 2 capsules, three times a day

Patient asked if she could eat, candy, gum, dark chocolate, ice cream and nuts. Also, could she have bacon and pork?

Answer: For nuts, only nut butter (such as hemp). No sugar or carbohydrates. Non-dairy ice cream is acceptable. No chocolate at this time. Natural sugars such as honey and stevia are allowed. Reinforced emphasis on all well-tolerated fruits, vegetables and proteins.

Fourth Appointment (2 weeks later):
Changes and additions/patient's progress and questions:

Progress: Diarrhea: stool is consistently formed (good news). Patient has more energy and is feeling stronger. Patient is not eating any junk food and is able to eat more vegetables and fruit.

Drug: Pentasa: Has reduced to five pills per day and will continue to reduce each week.

Addressing Abscess: Condition of abscess is yellow with white head that pops out. Extra protocol now involves blood purifying and destroying bacteria using herbal remedies. Refer to abscess and fistula segment further in this chapter, and the fifth appointment for liquid oxygen adjustment.

- L-Glutamine: 500 mg, once a day
- Liquid oxygen (internally): 7–9 drops and externally applied onto the abscess
- Magnesium citrate: 150 mg, twice a day

Patient's question: May I eat 70 percent organic chocolate, organic cocoa, Chinese food, string beans and tofu?

Answer: Organic chocolate is acceptable in small amounts, if tolerated. Tofu can be eaten, as well as Chinese food—with caution. String beans, if they can be digested.

Patient continues to progress. Her main problem currently is fistulas and abscess and on occasion, loose stools.

Fifth Appointment (2 weeks later):
Changes and additions/patient's progress and questions:

Progress: Crohn's symptoms continue to be stable even though antibiotics have been removed and the steady decrease of medication continues. The patient has yet to take the extra drug that was prescribed for her (Remicade) The patient is very happy with her progress and perspective future.

Drug: Pentasa: Patient has reduced to three pills per day and will continue to reduce each week.

Main Focus: Treating abscess and fistula. Stool requires bulking or firming up.

To firm up stool in colon, added 2 teaspoons psyllium husks in water, three times a day or more if desired, depending on its effectiveness. The psyllium husks will be added to the flaxseed mixture to be taken at mealtimes and once again at bedtime.

Abscess: Additional treatments prescribed:

- 1 cup of nettle and red clover tea, three times a day. This formula is for blood purifying and iron building.
- Poultice of slippery elm powder. Form a paste using aloe vera juice or gel. Add 2–3 drops of eucalyptus oil or lavender. Make a hot poultice and put on anal area for 15–20 minutes or until it has cooled. Heat again. Repeat two or three times a day if possible.
- Vitamin A/Beta-carotene: 30,000 IU once a day
- Vitamin E: 400 IU twice a day
- Oxygen drops: patient increased to 20 drops three times a day

Patient's complaint: Anti-viral formula is upsetting her stomach.

Answer: Take a small amount of yogurt first to coat the stomach. This is a good idea whenever nausea is a problem when taking pills or substances.

Sixth Appointment (2 weeks later):
Changes and additions/patient's progress and questions:

Progress: The patient is happy to be able to eat a healthy, more rounded diet. She is very pleased to see how much of a difference the diet "in and of itself" has made.

Drug: Pentasa: Has reduced to two pills per day and will continue to decrease. The patient is happy with her diet overall, since many foods that had presented a problem no longer cause adverse effects. *Type 'A' Crohn's disease patients will always have greater limitations than other gut disorder complaints.*

Main Focus: Treating fistula. Six months prior to this time, a rubber ring was surgically placed in through the fistula and another opening was made to accommodate the ring. The ring application was a repeated procedure. The patient had been told the ring would disintegrate before this time period, but it was uncomfortable and irritating. It has now been removed to enhance the healing process.

Example of Patient's Daily Eating Plan (Up Until This Point in Time)

Morning: 1 pint vegetable juice and 2 eggs with a small amount of hard cheese.

Lunch: Apples, almond butter, cheese, tofu pudding and cocoa (an approved product).

Dinner: Vegetable juice (if patient didn't have it at lunch). Quinoa or other tolerated grain-like food with cooked vegetables; fish or meat with vegetables. The patient is now adding a white potato occasionally at lunch time or when feeling hungry. I do not suggest food combining (starch and protein together at one meal). Food combining, which requires extra energy for the digestive system, is not advisable during a healing process.

Beverages: Herbal teas that are on the program; or, on occasion, a chocolate drink is permitted.

Other calming herbal teas would also be acceptable on this program; for example, chamomile, lemon balm, fennel, peppermint and anise. Choose herbs that are classified as antispasmodic or carminative for any gut discomfort.

Stool condition: Removed psyllium husks from the protocol. Stool has become too firm.

- Digestive enzyme combination (that also has pancreatic enzyme in the formula), one with each meal
- Proteolytic enzyme formula: reduced to 4 pills, three times a day on an empty stomach
- SAM-e: once per day
- Burdock root: 1 capsule, three times a day
- Teas, including red clover, ginger and peppermint

Patient's regular protocol remains the same.

Seventh Appointment (3 weeks later)
Changes and additions/patient's progress and questions

Progress: The abscess has healed a great deal.

Patient status: Patient is feeling really good at this time. Supplement and food regime is the same, with a bit more advice:

- Patient is eating quinoa, spelt, kamut and wild rice (black rice) with vegetables.
- I do not recommend that fruit such as dried apricots be mixed with dairy or grains.
- Berries and fruit that are permitted, including black berries, blueberries, cherries, coconut, gooseberries, mangos, papaya, pineapple, raspberries and strawberries.

TIP: Coconut helps with gas and some parasites. It also contains medium chained triglycerides (MCT's), as well as vitamin A, B1, B17, and D.

Drug: Pentasa has been reduced to 1 pill per day and will continue to reduce for one more week.

Change in Drug Protocol: Continuing drug elimination for two more consecutive weeks. Take one Pentasa pill every other day for the following two weeks, and then stop all Pentasa medication.

Eighth Appointment (4 weeks later):
Changes and additions/patient's progress and questions:

At 19 weeks, the patient has no Crohn's symptoms or complaints, and is off all medications.

Progress: Crohn's condition is stable with no symptoms or complaints at this time.

Drug Status: Patient is off all drugs and has been for the past 3 weeks. This is the state that all patients hope to reach for themselves.

Abscess and Fistula: For further healing effects, St. John's wort oil on a cotton pad prescribed (air is needed, so a Band Aid would be a problem). Additionally, clay packs are being applied to abscess and fistula area, which are helping. The program today is specifically geared at assisting the body in getting rid of the inflammation and infection in the anal area. The fistula opening is still there, although symptoms are much better; there's a little bit of improvement each day.

To further work on healing the opening and abscess, I continued to work on combating the bacteria in this area. The immune system is and continues to be strengthened by the ingestion of raw vegetable juices, colostrum, L-glutamine, vitamin A, zinc (and by not breaking the body down any further). By removing the offending substances like certain carbohydrates and sugars, the body can now begin its reversal process and commence healing itself.

Previous daily plan continues, with the following adjustments:
- Oregano oil and/or olive leaf oil: 2–3 drops, three times a day for two weeks. Then, reduce to 1 drop twice a day for destroying bacteria and viruses.
- Continue drinking red clover tea: 2 cups per day
- Raw garlic and fresh ginger added to food
- Burdock capsule: reduced from three times a day to twice a day

Surgeon suggestion: I recommended that patient see her surgeon about lancing or surgically removing the fistula openings that he had created. She is going to book an appointment. We should have an answer by her next appointment.

Ninth Appointment (4 weeks later):
Changes and additions /patient's progress and questions:

Patient's status: Crohn's symptoms have ceased for the past four months. The fistula is still healing slowly. The abscess has started to feel like it may want to drain again. A bit sorer, she reports. I am recommending an herb that destroys most microbes. Their life span is typically spread out over a three week period; therefore, four weeks will pick up any stragglers.

Hepatitis and Malaria shots: Patient is taking a holiday on an island where shots are recommended.

Previous daily plan continues, with the following adjustments:
- Black walnut hulls extract: dosage as directed, twice a day for 4 weeks
- Licorice DGL: 1–2 a day, as directed
- Slippery elm tea: 2 cups a day
- Flax seed tea enema: daily for one week

Tenth Appointment (4 weeks later):
Changes and additions/patient's progress and questions

Patient's status: Going on holiday. Taking licorice DGL to ensure digestion. Crohn's is still stable, with no urge to eliminate. Abscess is excreting a small amount of blood only for the last 5 days; no pus. There is a bulb that has formed in the abscess area. The body is cleansing impurities and so forth. I sent the patient to her doctor to have it lanced.

Previous daily plan continues, with the following adjustments:
- Protcolytic enzymes have been reduced to seven a day
- Hemp butter: for more protein and as snack
- Vitamin A capsule mixed with zinc oxide cream: to be used as a topical treatment on the abscess
- Stopped burdock root and yarrow tea
- Green tea loose leaf and ginger tea continues
- Juicing: dandelion to be added to each juice formula with watercress, every other day for two weeks
- Kale soup

Eleventh Appointment (4 weeks later):
Changes and additions/patient's progress and questions:

Patient status: Patient saw the surgeon, and lancing the abscess bulb in the anal area was not a problem. It healed up nicely. The patient reported that her rectum area and gut are no longer sore and no diarrhea. She went on her holiday, had a great time and is going back. Diet on her holiday consisted of vegetables, fruit, protein and some form of dessert.

Note: Seven months in, and the patient is still not consuming any other carbohydrates.

Twelfth Appointment (9 weeks later):
Changes and additions/patient's progress and questions:

Gastroenterologist: Patient visited her specialist and proceeded to tell him that she no longer has any Crohn's symptoms. He then asked if she had taken the new medication (Remicade) that was prescribed. She told him that she had instead taken the natural approach and seen a holistic doctor and was off all of her medications for a month. She asked if he had any other suggestions; his reply was, "No, just keep doing what you are doing."

This patient will continue with her normal restricted diet, while some of the supplements will be reduced or cancelled. The abscess area still needs to be addressed, even though the healing process has accelerated, with the following changes:

- Colloidal silver: internally as directed, plus externally at night time only, on a pad or gauze fitted over the abscess area.
- Continue to clean the blood for another six months using sage and red clover tea, alternately consuming 2 cups sage and 1 cup red clover, reversing every second day.
- Proteolytic enzymes will continue for two more months, taking one pill three times a day for the first month, and reducing one pill a day until finished.

For further information, refer to the patient update at the end of the summary.

Summary of Case History: Type 'A' Crohn's Disease Patient

This patient came to me with extremely severe symptoms and complications of Crohn's disease. Her symptoms included constant diarrhea, bleeding, fistula with a surgically implanted ring, anal abscesses, no energy, low libido, mild depression and great difficulty finding something to eat that didn't trigger the diarrhea and gas. Her diet consisted of starches, carbohydrates, sugar products (as she had a sweet tooth), protein, dairy, decaffeinated coffee, soda (occasionally), and virtually no vegetables or fruit. Her drug plan included antibiotics twice a day and two pills of Pentasa four times a day. In an attempt to find further healing, she went for twenty hours of hyperbaric oxygen treatments (HBOT). She experienced a 15 percent healing and had less pain in her rectum area.

Hyperbaric Oxygen Treatment (HBOT)

The following is a brief explanation about HBOT application:

Under normal conditions, 97.5 percent of oxygen is carried in the blood-stream bound to hemoglobin, with the remaining 2.5 percent is dissolved in plasma. Traditional uses of hyperbaric oxygen treatment (HBOT) include treating decompression sickness, air embolisms, carbon monoxide poisoning, acute traumatic ischemia (crush injuries that deprive tissues of oxygen), and bacterial invasions of a necrotic wound (tissue has died).

Today, HBOT is a technique used to deliver 100 percent oxygen directly to an open, moist wound. Topical HBOT oxygen device consists of an appliance to enclose the wound area (frequently an extremity) and a source of oxygen (conventional oxygen tanks may be used). Topical HBOT has been explored as a treatment of skin ulcerations due to diabetes, venous stasis, post-surgical infection, gangrenous lesion, decubitus ulcers, amputation, skin graft, burns or frostbite.

I quickly determined that the patient's gut symptoms were not consistent with a typical inflammatory bowel disorder, especially since her rectum area had degenerated to such a large degree. Her condition included a fistula with a surgically implanted ring, a repeated procedure in her treatment history performed by her gastroenterologist. Diarrhea with bleeding occurred five to six times a day. Many people who have Crohn's disease and colitis are mainly just gluten (and sometimes dairy) intolerant. Corn may produce intermittent reactions, as well as a few other common irritants. This case is an example of someone who has an inability to digest sugars properly, throughout the intestinal tract. If these foods were not such a threat, her body would not have responded in the way that it did. The patient experienced a rapid reversal in her Crohn's symptoms within 4–8 weeks, showing us both that the recommended treatment plan was working effectively. By the end of the fourth month, the patient was completely drug-free and has remained so.

The first step was to build her body up on all levels; in particular, her immune and endocrine systems. We also needed to effect a complete change in her daily diet routine. Most of the foods she had been eating were taken away, and others were introduced in a form that was tolerated bearing in mind her current digestive capabilities. The patient immediately responded favorably to her new regime. She didn't have any nausea from her recommended supplements or the foods she was eating. The diet needed to be very light on the digestive system to start a healing process of this nature. Raw fluids are best assimilated and nourishing at this time. Broths made from beef bones are helpful as well, so long as they include the marrow and joint material, as they are body building and easily digested.

The treatment plan involved a great deal more work and due diligence on the part of the patient than would have been otherwise required with a more common Crohn's or ulcerative colitis complaint. This patient showed complete compliance with the diet changes and restrictions. Because of these modifications, she and I were rewarded with a quick healing response. The work that remained involved healing the fistula and abscess. This type of problem involves much more than the actual location of the infection or problem. In these related types of cases, the blood and immune system need to be addressed. This is accomplished by purifying the blood using herbal remedies, mainly in the form of teas and tinctures (and sometimes capsule form). Herbal remedies were again called upon to replace antibiotics to rid the body of the pathogens that can lead to infection and inflammation. Note that trials still continue in an endeavor to heal the abscess and fistula.

Great strides were made in restoring the tissue integrity of the rectum area. The patient reached a point where she no longer had pain or discomfort in the anal area. However, the fistula had been a long time problem, causing a ring or cord to be surgically inserted on more than one occasion. The fistula also presented a problem due to the ring and its time duration, which had formed scar tissue much like a piercing for earrings. The abscess next to this area resembled a painful boil. The complete healing of this area will require time and effort on the part of the patient, as she continues to apply the compresses and so forth on a regular basis to assist the healing process. Unless the surgeon considers minimizing the holes that were opened for drainage, I am not confident that they will close up completely; only time will tell. For the most part, the abscess is under control, but little flare-ups still occur on occasion. The patient continues to work at reversing any remaining symptoms and in preventing any previous ones from returning by empowering the body to heal itself.

The benefits, when observed from the patient's point of view, are enormous. By working through the cause of their complaint, they were able to:

- Renew their health
- Their future health prospects are much brighter
- Restored a semblance of normalcy in their everyday life
- A great deal of fear is removed when away from the house
- Enhanced quality of personal and family life
- Eating has become pleasurable and safe
- Alertness provided by increased knowledge if symptoms arise in another family member indicating inherited weakness
- Increased energy
- Zest for life has returned; now entertaining new ideas or options
- No more pain from gut symptoms
- No more symptoms of diarrhea, gas, nausea or bloating
- No more medications
- No more frequent doctor office visits
- No more expensive medical costs (for those who do not have medical coverage)

So, the next time you hear that Crohn's disease and other similar complaints are incurable, or that you will always require surgery, you should remember that there is an alternative choice. Gut disorders have a strong association with the foods and substances that we take into our bodies. Mainstream medicine does not have a vested interest in dealing with the cause of many disorders. Allopathic doctors treat the symptoms only, which typically involve many office visits, expensive medications, surgery and, unfortunately, the progression of the disease. When taking an alternative approach, the patient is fully involved with the healing process and maintenance of their condition.

UPDATE (2015): Crohn's Type 'A' Patient

Since I haven't had any contact with the patient in the last several years, I was wondering how the healing of her abscesses had progressed. On January 8, 2015, I contacted the patient to get an update. To my surprise, her abscesses have completely healed, including the openings made by the surgically repeated rubber ring insertion.

A Common Diet-Related Colitis Case History

The patient in this case had a long history of gut complaints, which have now been diagnosed as colitis. Her treatment thus far through her G.I. specialist and her family's general practitioner has been, at best, far less than adequate. I have counseled her three times over the past two years. I removed items from her diet, such as gluten products like bread and caffeinated beverages, fats, sugar products, chocolate, oranges and other related food items.

I felt we needed to find out more about any specific allergies she might have. She went for an ELISA/ACT test (an enzyme linked immunosorbent assay advanced cell test). This is a special blood test that measures circulating antibody levels to as many as 300 foods and chemicals. Candida can also be determined by the ELISA/ACT test, while parasitic infections can be diagnosed by stool analysis or rectal swabs. The test showed she was allergic to the nightshade family—peppers, potatoes, eggplant, and tomatoes. She is also gluten-sensitive and lactose-intolerant.

The patient lost 25 pounds in the first four months (mainly from removing all flour ingredients that have gluten). She makes steady improvement as long as she adheres to her regimen; at times when she doesn't, there is no mistaking it. Her body reacts very quickly, as do most people with intestinal disorders.

Supplements recommended: chlorella, zinc, calcium, magnesium, B-complex with extra B12, aloe vera gel, flax seed tea, comfrey tea, vitamin E, folic acid, vitamin A-beta carotene, non-acidic fruits and vegetables, psyllium husks and vegetable juicing.

This patient turned her life around by changing her diet. Besides losing stubborn, unwanted pounds, she exhibited a renewed interest in her appearance, career and personal happiness and health.

Patient Testimonial

Patient Name: "Jill"
Date: August 2012

I have had stomach issues all my life. After each meal, discomfort, bloating, pain were ever present...it was my "normal." Through my forties, things got much worse with an inability to process most foods, ongoing bouts of severe diarrhea, significant weight loss, a decrease in mental acuity, and the presence of abscesses and development of a fistula. The auto-immune response I experienced meant my body was riddled with arthritis and my joints were swollen and painful all the time. I sought advice from allopathic doctors, medical intuitives, energy healers, naturopaths and homeopaths with no noticeable improvement in health. In some cases, treatment even exacerbated the problems. A colo-rectal surgeon actually suggested exploratory surgery and thought a colostomy might be needed.

Then a friend referred me to Michelle Honda. I had not yet seen a holistic doctor, so I made an appointment. After my earlier experiences with health care practitioners, I had low expectations and little hope that she would be able to help. My first meeting with Michelle was a thorough, two hour non-invasive "examination"—otherwise known as a discussion. We talked about the root causes of my issues and what was happening in my body. She recommended an alkaline diet, juicing, herbal teas, herbal sitz baths (and enema) and supplements. What did I have to lose? I bought everything I needed and started the treatment program. Within 48 hours, all auto-immune symptoms had disappeared. For the first time in my life, I was pain free. I could eat and process food without any discomfort.

'Is this how most people feel?' I thought. What a new experience for me. I started redefining "normal". My mental sharpness returned and I began to feel smart again. I had an abundance of energy. Whereas in the past I would accept social invitations tentatively, as I never knew how I would be feeling on any given day, now my social calendar is full and I am making up for lost time! My dream had always been to visit Africa, but I never thought I would be able to venture that far from home, considering my health issues. Thanks to Michelle, that no longer concerns me. I leave for Kenya and Tanzania next month!

Cheers!
Jill

UPDATE (2015): Jill's Current Health Status

Jill's health remained superb. She had long had desire to go to Africa, but had put the trip off due to persistent unstable health symptoms. Jill did go to Kenya and Tanzania as planned and had a great time. She recently took a trip to India, where long trips far away from familiar medial practices would have delayed her travel.

Jill has not taken her renewed health status for granted. She continues with a healthy eating regime that includes vegetable juicing and a supplement maintanence program.

All of which is just another example of the power within the body to heal itself, so long as it is supported and given a chance.

CASE HISTORY: Crohn's Disease/Fistula (2015)
Following the Quick Start Program

The following case history is an example of a patient who followed the Quick Start Program over five weeks. This is a more complicated case of Crohn's, and yet the turn around is remarkable.

Health History

On January 8, 2015, a young male, 15 years of age, accompanied by his parents came to me presenting with Crohn's disease and complications of anal fistula, and had recently experienced rapid weight loss (current weight: 105 pounds). Other symptoms consisted of diarrhea, bleeding, stomach pain, and fatigue.

Upon first meeting the patient, I initially observed dark circles under his eyes, with a clearly visible lack of energy and an overall weakened state.

From my dialogue with the patient's parents, I determined the culprit of his illness to be the result of a trip to a Caribbean island, where he either experienced food poisoning or foreign bacteria (parasites did not show up in testing). The patient was diagnosed with Crohn's disease in 2011, with scars showing on his terminal ileum. The anal fistula had been a constant presence for 18 months prior to this first appointment. Near the end of October, into November 2014, the patient lost approximately 12 pounds in one week. Dairy has also been a problem since the age of 10.

The patient's past medication history initially included antibiotics and corticosteroids, which were followed by immunosuppressant drugs. When these did not work, they then moved on to a few others in subsequent order: budersonide, infliximab, and then methotexate and remicade taken together (which started in 2013). Remicade started out at 8-week intervals and increased to every four weeks, and yet the young man was still getting worse.

His mother had been removing carbs, gluten, and dairy from her son's diet since November 2014, but symptoms still persisted. The problem stems from the fact that medications interfere with normal body functions and therefore can either directly interfere with the healing process *or* they can slow it down.

Current Medications

The patient had been taking two medications: Remicade (300 ml) and Metronidazole (250 mg once a week). He was experiencing diarrhea even though he was not scheduled for another Remicade session for five more weeks. The time interval between Remicade treatments has been systematically shortened to try to accommodate his returning symptoms of diarrhea and bleeding. The patient's diet has also become very limited. Previous testing involved an endoscopy and an MRI.

First Appointment: Initiating the Quick Start Program

With the assistance of the patient's mother, the young man started my Quick Start Program, as detailed in Chapter 5.

The herb agrimony tincture is suggested for episodes of diarrhea and bleeding. This is normally an initial recommendation, but as the diarrhea wasn't severe, I suggested waiting until symptoms showed up that would warrant its usage. It is possible for sufficient healing to take place without the use of multiple remedies. This would also tell me how well his body is responding on its own, and demonstrate to the parents whether or not the medications can start being reduced.

The patient was to take most of the supplements suggested in the Quick Start Program, since his body was severely lacking in adequate nutrition. The intake of my vegetable juice formula was to be drunk twice a day until sufficient healing progress had been made. (See the patient's supplemental program and how it benefited him further on in this case history.)

The patient was not local to the area and had decided to order the comfrey root online, which they received within a few days. Once the comfrey root became available, the patient was to drink three cups per day, mixed with equal amounts of slippery elm. The same tea mixture was to be administered in the form of a retention enema daily for the treatment of the fistula, as well as for direct healing to the surface of the sigmoid and descending colon region.

Second Follow-Up Appointment: Two Weeks Later

It has been two weeks since last contact with the patient. Immediately upon seeing the patient I observed a remarkable difference. He had a wide smile and the circles under his eyes were gone. He reported having a lot more energy and was able to eat a larger quantity of food. Bowel movements have been reduced to only two a day—in the morning before school and in the evening after dinner. The fistula has even started to close. The parents were very surprised to see such a drastic change in their son in such a short amount of time.

My initial concern for this patient, like others who are current students, was his being in a classroom and having to leave during class. Normally just thinking about, "Will I have to leave the room during class?" is enough to bring about a sense of urgency, requiring a visit to the bathroom. But surprisingly, this did not happen. I applaud his parents for following through on all of my recommendations, and for the compliance on the part of the patient.

- During the two week period since I first met the patient, he had administered the retention enemas 11 of the 14 days. The fistula had already started to close.
- He drank three cups of tea per day. The patient actually liked the tea.
- The patient took supplements as recommended.
- The patient consumed one pint of vegetable juice three times a day (when possible): before school, in the afternoon and in the evening, a couple hours after dinner.

The Patient's Diet for the Past Two Weeks

The young man was able to eat lots of gluten-free grains; therefore, he does not need to be on a carbohydrate-free diet. The patient *did* ask if he could eat smoked salmon; I advised him not to eat it for the time being, and to avoid as many food chemicals as possible. Also, I recommended that he not food combine (starch and protein at one mealtime). The diet was geared around easily digested foods, in the form of soup and juices, until there were no longer any symptoms. If so, he could eat small amounts of solid food.

Drug Metronidazole

Because the patient's symptoms were under control, I gave the parents the option to reduce the dosage of the drug metronidazole. This was also to test whether any symptoms might show up.

Protocol

The protocol remained the same until our next visit. I recommended waiting until it was close to the time-frame for repeating the drug Remicade, which was three weeks away, before our next meeting. I did not adjust or add any more remedies. So far, the herb agrimony was not needed.

Third Appointment: Three Weeks Later

The patient's weight is up to 118 pounds. The parents have completely stopped the drug Metronidazole, declaring that absolutely no unwanted symptoms had returned and that he is much stronger. The fistula has been fully closed for one month with exception to one day, where there had been a small amount of leakage, after which it had remained closed. The astringent herb argimony for diarrhea and bleeding was not required. The protocol is to remain the same until the fistula is well healed. Soon the enemas may be reduced to 3–4 a week, and then fewer as time goes on, and can eventually be stopped altogether. As long as healing continues without any symptom reoccurrence, the tea can be reduced to two cups per day.

The father wanted a return visit in two weeks time. However, since there were no symptoms for me to work on, I suggested waiting 6–8 weeks, at which time a reduction in protocol, supplements and so forth could be put in place.

The patient and family both realized the importance of health maintenance by way of thyroid care and supplements like fish oil, probiotics, raw juices, and minerals for extra insurance. I stressed the importance of avoiding gluten and any irritating substances for at least one year, even though the patient may feel great.

The credit for the rapid turnaround falls solely upon the parents and the patient. This scenario is what I refer to as the Fast Track. I never cease to be amazed by what is possible when the body as a whole is enhanced and properly supported. The main point to note here is that during the initial stage, when the greatest amount of effort is applied *in the short term,* evidence will provide the hope and discipline for a better future—one that is far sooner than later.

Vacation in April 2015

During the patient's last appointment, I was informed that they are taking a vacation in approximately six weeks time. I recommended the whole family take 1 teaspoon of colloidal silver daily while away for insurance against infection and pathogens (especially for the patient).

Medications Fall Away

It has only been five weeks since the patient started the program and yet so much progress has been made. From this case history, you can see how medications become unneeded and unhelpful. Notice that I did not need to recommend antibiotic replacements or alternative remedies to destroy widespread pathogens. My recommendation was not to repeat any medications.

Supplement Breakdown

Fish Oil: Fish oil was the only remedy for inflammation prescribed, and was performing multiple duties. Inflammation is reduced by the healing properties in the herbal tea blend as tissue repair continues (1000 mg, three times a day).

Colostrum: Colostrum was instrumental in boosting the patient's immune system and enhancing the healing process (900 mg, twice a day).

L-glutamine: L-glutamine increased intestinal cell replication and boosted moods and the immune system (500 mg, three times a day).

Vegetable Juice: The antioxidants in the vegetable juice formula also helped with inflammation and covered a great deal of nutrition and electrolyte requirements (2 cups twice a day).

Endocrine Support: Initially, supporting the thyroid and adrenals provided the quickest turn-around in energy uptake, along with vegetable juicing (L-tyrosine 500 mg, 1–2 times a day, and iodine drops as directed by the product of choice). In addition, I recommended glandular desiccated extract in a combination formula for all other glands and organs (two capsules twice a day).

Minerals: Zinc and magnesium are necessary for metabolic functions and their designated duties. Magnesium can be crucial to the healing process for Crohn's disease and ulcerative colitis (Magnesium citrate 300 mg, three times a day and zinc 25 mg, twice a day).

Nutritional Flaked Yeast: A complete protein source, nutritional flaked yeast contains all B vitamins. B vitamins and amino acids that are used heavily throughout the body (1 tablespoon twice a day).

B12: B12 is often required in cases of Crohn's disease and ulcerative colitis. The absorption of this vitamin is greatly compromised when the ileum is affected by these diseases (1200 mcg once a day, under the tongue).

Liquid Chlorophyll: The patient sipped liquid chlorophyll throughout the day in water to boost minerals, iron levels, and for its soothing and alkalizing effects (1–2 teaspoons of concentrate in an eight ounce glass of water).

Probiotics: Friendly flora are required to rebalance the intestines and large colon with beneficial bacteria and reduce the overall population of harmful microbes in these regions. It is also required by the thyroid gland for functioning, and plays a role in our immune system (Commercial acidophilus and bifidus supplement, two capsules twice a day).

Vitamin D: Vitamin D has Crohn's disease inhibiting effects and anti-microbial benefits (2000 IU twice a day).

Vitamin E: Used for its antioxidant and anti-scarring benefits (400 IU three times a day).

Flax Seed Oil: Used for additional omega-3 fatty acids (1 tablespoon twice a day).

Herbal Teas: Quickens repair of intestinal tissue, and is also highly instrumental in reducing the symptoms of diarrhea, bleeding and inflammation throughout the whole GI tract (Comfrey root and slippery elm bark in equal parts using the decoction process, one cup 3 times a day).

Enemas: Retention enemas provide accelerated healing and soothing for inflamed colon tissue. They help heal fistulas and abscesses more quickly.

The same tea mixture described above was administered as an enema daily during the evening, and held for 30 minutes. Since the colon is an extremely acidic area, it becomes harder to relieve inflammation and heal lesions. The tea in the retention enema provides direct and speedier healing to the surface of the large colon and rectal area.

Agrimony: While the herb agrimony was *not* required, it will be useful if any incident in the future shows up, either from eating a forbidden food or from harmful pathogens. Even though enormous progress has been made, newly healed tissue requires time to strengthen, as does the whole body.

Last Appointment: 10 Weeks Later
Today's appointment centers on the patient's recent diet and any changes made to his daily regimen since our last contact. A main focus for this appointment is the elimination and reduction of supplements and protocols, such as the retention enemas.

The patient and his parents are extremely happy with the disease's reversal. His current weight is now 133 pounds. The vacation took place two weeks ago, without any returning symptoms. The fistula has remained closed. All the previous recommendations have been adhered to, with light exception during the vacation, where there was a slight reduction.

Even though there have not been any Crohn's disease symptoms or complications, I still consider this time-frame to be the early stages of healing. The newly formed tissue requires further development and strengthening, and there may be remnants of intestinal tract lesions that are not fully healed.

The main concern is to be extremely careful for several months, making sure to eat only what is tolerated. A few days prior to this appointment, the patient's mother purchased a high-quality cream cheese from her special yogurt distributor. As noted in the patient's health history, he had not been able to tolerate dairy for many years prior to his Crohn's disease condition. Because the product was of a higher quality, the mother did not think about the difference in the ingredients that make up these two products. I was actually happy that he had experienced one occurrence of diarrhea, to demonstrate how sensitive the body has become to anything that presents itself as an antigen or an intolerant substance. Because they had not needed to use the agrimony for diarrhea previously, they took this opportunity to sample how it works. The mother reported that it stopped the diarrhea very quickly.

Most of the appointment involved reinforcing the responsibility the patient has regarding what he consumes for the next 6–12 months. A problem stems from the fact that he feels so great, being medication-free with his body functions normal. For the foreseeable future, when he is eating out or when someone else is feeding him, he must know to ask whether the food is safe for him to eat. In the case of this patient, he may be able to reintroduce gluten in 1–2 years but for any known intolerance, such as dairy in his case, avoidance is best.

Current and Future Supplement Regimen

Vegetable juice: Continue at 1 pint twice a day for two more weeks, before reducing to once a day, preferably in the morning.

Healing tea: Drink 1 cup three times a day for two more weeks, and then reduce to 1 cup twice a day for six weeks, and then stop. Otherwise, reduce to 1 cup a day for one month more per their discretion.

Retention enemas: Reduced to five times a week for four more weeks to ensure the fistula is well-healed on the inside of the rectum wall, before stopping.

Fish oil: 1000 mg, twice a day ongoing for normal health maintenance.

L-Glutamine: 500 mg, twice a day for two more months, and then stop.

Colostrum: 900 mg, twice a day for two more months, and then stop.

Endocrine Support: Desiccated glandular extract: 1 capsule twice a day. Continue this dosage for the next three months and then reducing to one a day.

Thyroid Maintenance: Iodine drops daily and one 500 mg L-Tyrosine once a day. The tyrosine may be reduced to 3–5 times a week in the future unless his lifestyle starts to become stressful or from overworking for prolonged periods of time.

Magnesium: 300 mg, twice a day for several months and then reduce to once a day for health maintenance.

Zinc: 25 mg, twice a day for two more weeks, and then reduce to once a day unless a cold or other infection occurs in the future, at which point increase to twice a day, until feeling well and returning to once a day.

Probiotics: Two capsules twice a day for one year, and then as the brand suggests for health maintenance. Once the microbes are well-balanced in the intestinal tract, 3–5 times a week for maintaining future bacterium balance is normally sufficient. Even missing a few weeks at a time while on a vacation will not present a problem, unless you are currently suffering from intestinal disease symptoms.

Vitamin D: 1000 mg, twice a day for six months. Future recommendation: 1000 mg, once a day, and 1000 mg, twice a day during the winter months.

This case history is for people who are all-too-often told that diet has nothing to do with their disease; that it does not make any difference what you eat and that you will never be able to stop your medications. Another (false) statement I often hear repeated by my patients is that nothing natural will work. These case histories are just a few examples of the restorative power inside whole, unadulterated food and complementary medicine.

CHAPTER SEVEN

Replace Popular Medications with Safe and Effective Natural Alternatives

Natural Alternatives to Popular Pain Medication

Pain affects more North Americans than any other disorder. Natural healing therapies work to relieve pain by calming the nerves and increasing circulation, promoting healing without suppressing the condition. Natural therapies include the use of enzymes, amino acids, minerals and Cyclooxygenase (COX-2) inhibiting herbs. (Cyclooxygenase (COX) is an enzyme, officially identified as prostaglandin-endoperoxide synthase (PTGS). The abbreviation "COX" is seen throughout medical literature as an indicator for inhibiting the pathways of pain and inflammation.) Today, many herbs are being reported to possess COX-2 inhibiting properties, which have long since been used by ancient medical traditions.

Pain is also a common symptom that plagues those suffering from gastrointestinal disorders. The degree of pain varies, and can range from a mild ache due to bloating and cramping to a debilitating, life-altering level of pain. Another type of pain, which causes severe discomfort, is felt as a sharp stabbing pain or a dull achy pain, which increases to an intense pain in waves and involves nausea and vomiting.

The main focus in treating gut pain is reducing inflammation, preferably through natural options. As evidential studies have shown that bacterial infection may be the culprit linked to the inflammation, there must also be a focus on dealing with any and all pertinent infections. Refer to "Natural Alternatives for Antibiotics and Destroying Superbugs" later in this chapter for substances that kill bacteria and antibiotic resistant superbugs.

The issue with anti-inflammatory drugs is that, while they have demonstrated short-term effects in reducing pain, they can become ineffective over time and can even lead to steroid dependency. In addition, medications normally prescribed for inflammation and immune system suppression can actually cause flare-ups in many people, while other complications of prescription medications include heightened blood pressure and osteoporosis.

Inflammation is linked to free radical formation, and is associated with degenerative diseases and aging. The link between antioxidants and inflammation is that antioxidants *kill* free radicals. By adjusting our diet to include foods high in antioxidants, our body's inflammatory responses are dampened. Foods of particular benefit include green tea, fish oils, wild fish, dark colored vegetables, and fruits (such as cherries and red, blue and blackberries). Some herbs are especially useful, as they possess both anti-inflammatory and antioxidant properties, such as can be found in garlic, onions, ginger, chives, rosemary, turmeric, oregano and basil. Pectin (found in apples and some citrus fruits) has been shown to reduce or eliminate arthritis symptoms and to improve the health of veins, arteries and connective tissue.

Pain interferes with our daily enjoyment of life. Many herbs containing anti-inflammatory properties frequently possess very powerful antiviral, antibacterial and even anti-pathogenic substances. This in effect means that both the inflammation and its cause are being dealt with at the same time. For this reason, herbs are very successful in remedying inflammatory conditions. Alternative health care practitioners employ a wide range of complementary therapies and techniques to treat an individual's pain. They can also provide therapeutic dosages.

Phellodendron Bark (*Phellodendron amurense*) **extract** not only has COX-2 inhibiting qualities, but also helps protect the gastrointestinal tract against ulceration. It will even protect the stomach lining when you are using NSAIDs and conventional COX-2 inhibitors.

Suggested dosage for gut inflammation:

- Dried powder: 3–10 grams per day
- 4:1 dried decoction: 1–3 grams per day
- Other pain, including joint pain: 300 mg capsules, taken 2–3 times per day

Relora: Magnolia and **Phellodendron** go well together. Both of these herbs have a lineage for reducing pain and inflammation throughout the body.

Suggested dosage: 250–500 mg, taken twice a day with meals

Turmeric (*Curcuma Iongo*) is an herb valued for its anti-inflammatory properties, which are due to a chemical called curcumin, which research has reported to be a powerful COX-2 inhibitor. Turmeric root is traditionally used in Chinese and Ayurvedic medicine for inflammatory conditions, as well as a wide range of other disorders.

Suggested dosage: 500 mg, 3–6 times a day, coupled with 200 mg of **Bromelain** to enhance effectiveness.

Boswellia, also known as frankincense, has been shown in studies to be helpful for both rheumatoid and osteoarthritis with the pain index falling by 90 percent after eight weeks, with an equally dramatic increase in function. Boswellia is an effective remedy for ulcerative colitis and other inflammatory conditions. Similarly to phellodendron bark, boswellia doesn't appear to cause the gut irritation that can occur with many conventional pain medications. The resin extracted from the boswellia tree also has significant anti-inflammatory properties, and is beneficial for asthma, irritable bowel syndrome, Crohn's disease and other painful complaints.

A 1997 study of individuals with ulcerative colitis found that 82 percent of those who took boswellia extract (350 milligrams, three times daily) experienced remission. Rare side effects of boswellia include diarrhea, nausea and skin rash.

Suggested dosage for inflammation: 500 mg, 3–5 times per day

White willow bark (*Salix alba*) contains natural salicylic acid, the active component in aspirin. Many studies have been done on this plant's unique property, and they consistently show its effectiveness in reducing pain. For example, in two studies of 661 patients with chronic severe lower back pain, 240 mg of white willow bark extract left 40 percent of patients pain-free after four weeks, with improvement evident after only one week of treatment. In those receiving standard orthopedic care and Motrin for 4 weeks, only 18 percent were pain free. There were no adverse effects on the stomach lining from the white willow bark. Furthermore, white willow bark benefits Crohn's disease, ulcerative colitis, ulcers, irritable bowel syndrome and many other conditions characterized by pain and inflammation.

Suggested dosage: As needed, 500 mg or ½ teaspoon powder taken often for acute symptoms. Decrease as improvement is felt. Take as tea in a decoction process.

Holy Basil (*Ocimum sanctum*) contains phytochemicals that have COX-2 inhibiting effects. In Egypt, this herb is traditionally used for arthritis and inflammation. French researchers have shown it to be a potent COX-2 inhibitor, while studies performed in other nations around the world have confirmed these findings. Since holy basil has been shown to possess potent anti-inflammatory properties, it lends itself well to the treatment of gut and stomach ulcers, as well as bowel inflammation complaints, including irritable bowel syndrome.

Suggested dosage: 500 mg, 3–6 times per day

Glucosamine is a building block for connective tissues like cartilage and collagen. Since the publication of *The Arthritis Cure* in 1996, a large number of people began to treat their joint pain with glucosamine sulfate rather than NASIDs, and reported their findings to their physicians. Subjectively, 75–80 percent of people reported drastic improvement in their pain and mobility. The Rheumatic Disease Unit at Queen's University has done numerous clinical studies on "glucosamine sulfate and osteoarthritis." The report states that, "Overall, glucosamine sulfate was found to be safe and effective in treating arthritis." Another possible consideration is glucosamine hydrochloride. Glucosamine is a large molecule that is hard to absorb. Check for the type and form that best enhances absorbability. Take as directed or double up on the dosage, divided up throughout the day.

Collagen is known as the "glue in life," functioning as a protective agent for cartilage and synovial fluid against deterioration. Cartilage consists of 67 percent collagen. Oral collagen has been shown to improve joint mobility, reduce pain, regenerate cartilage and muscle and promote tissue recovery. Sleep is a necessity to enable the body to repair and utilize collagen. During REM sleep, the body converts available collagen and other nutrients into new tissue. For best results when consuming supplemental collagen, take on an empty stomach at bedtime.

Suggested dosage: 1000 mg, once per day. May also be combined with Hyluronic acid for extra support.

Amino acids have proven useful in treating pain, allergies and depression and in reducing inflammation in patients with chronic pain disorders. The amino acid DL-Phenylalanine can raise the body's threshold for pain and sensitivity by effectively releasing the body's own natural pain killers, known as endorphins. This amino acid also inhibits the breakdown of endorphins, while converting chemicals in the brain which elevate mood, relieving depression.

Suggested dosage: 1000 mg, 2–3 times a day. Also consider an amino acid complex formula.

Enzymes (in the form of supplementation) aid digestion and absorption and reduce or eliminate pain. Bromelain, a pineapple extract, is an anti-inflammatory enzyme often seen being coupled with pain-relieving herbs like turmeric. Other beneficial uses of bromelain include being used as a blood pressure reducing agent, heart and stroke inhibitor and a healing accelerator.

Mangosteen taken in supplement form has been found to relieve symptoms of pain, inflammation and diarrhea for those with inflammatory bowel disorder (IBD) and other similar gut complications. Scientific research has shown mangosteen to possess COX-2 inhibiting properties, but does not inhibit the production of Cyclooxygenase (COX-1) enzymes.

Suggested dosage: 500 mg, taken 2–3 times per day. Beverages are dosed from 1–2 ounces (30–60 ml) 2–3 times a day.

Natural Alternatives for Antibiotics and Destroying Superbugs

It is crucial for all gut disorder patients to be vigilant in protecting themselves against all infection. Persons with gut dysbiosis are already at a disadvantage, because they have an overworked immune system and gut permeability. Enhancing your immune response is a primary focus in your defense against bacteria. A strategic way to halt aggressive bugs is through immune system support and thorough meticulous cleansing of the body and wounds with gentle antibacterial soaps, to cripple MRSA and other staph colonization.

Can Antibiotics Cause Crohn's Disease and Colitis?

News reports have shown that people who have consumed large quantities of antibiotics tend to be at a higher risk of inflammatory bowel disease (IBD). A supportive study demonstrating antibiotic abuse was published in the American Journal of Gastroenterology. Based on a sample of more than 24,000 people, the study indicated that the use of antibiotics can disturb the normal "friendly" bacteria balance in the gut. From previous studies, all severe gut disorders, including Crohn's disease and ulcerative colitis, were linked to antibiotics. Dramatic reports are continuing to surface showing that antibiotics are solely responsible for people contracting conditions of inflammatory bowel disease (IBD). For example, a study report detailed cases where antibiotics were exclusively responsible for IBD: *Every 20 people prescribed three or more antibiotics resulted in one additional case of inflammatory bowel disease.*

Throughout the UK and North America, the statistics are not looking any better. As researchers gathered other factors into account, they found that people taking repetitive antibiotic prescriptions were 50 percent more likely to get Crohn's disease within 2–5 years. In recounting all of these aspects, some scientists think conditions such as Crohn's disease and ulcerative colitis (IBD) may result from the immune system overreacting to viruses or bacteria in the intestine. Together, these two diseases are thought to affect approximately 1 in every 250 people in the UK.

Worldwide Concern of Antibiotic Overuse (WHO Agency Report)

The World Health Organization (WHO) has collaborated with other member states and affiliates over the ever-increasing instances of viruses, parasites and bacterium becoming antimicrobial resistant (AMR). Globally, the overuse of antibiotics has created a worldwide concern. The agency stated, "Without urgent action, we are heading for a post-antibiotic era, in which common infections and minor injuries can once again kill."

There has never been such a great need for effective treatment as in this present time. The logical choice is to return to the curative plants and substances that nature provides. As has been (and will continue to be) demonstrated in this book, nature does indeed hold the solution to this problem.

How Do Patients Protect Themselves from Harmful and Deadly Germs?

An alternative solution to antibiotics is required to combat the different varieties of microbes a person may routinely be exposed to in daily life. Another concern is the person's internal microbial environment, which can be causing pain, inflammation and diarrhea. The latter is often the reason for the antibiotic prescription in the first place. For the remainder of this chapter, we'll be examining the major concerns of superbugs and how to eradicate unwanted bacteria—*without* the use of antibiotics.

The Hospital Visit
Today, an environment such as a hospital is no longer the safe haven it once was. While visiting medical clinics or during an extended hospital stay, patients must now struggle to stay healthy while being treated for an entirely different disorder. The bacterium strain Methicillin Resistant Staphylococcus (MRSA) and C-defficile are responsible for the rise of many difficult-to-treat infections in humans. Our new awareness in this area has curbed our use of antibiotics. Research has found that different strains of bacteria such as C-defficile, MRSA and other superbugs can actually survive by consuming antibiotics "alone." Since many patients with bowel disorders of varying natures have been exposed to unsafe environments such as hospitals and doctor's offices, having knowledge of alternative substances to replace antibiotics may be crucial. Further complicating matters is the fact that these individuals have had repeated prescriptions of antibiotics which also reduces their effectiveness.

Antibiotic Replacements That Are Safe and Effective

New strategies and alternative approaches have become necessary to destroy and prevent recurring infections from superbugs and staph bacterium. There are a number of natural remedies available to treat antibiotic resistant bacteria with highly successful results while still being cost effective. Do not limit these remedies to superbugs; consider natural alternatives any time the body requires a healing agent involving inflammation and infection. The following natural solutions are a perfect choice to help with the healing process and symptoms of gut pain and inflammation.

General Protocol

Initially, upon suspicion of C-deffcile, noro virus or MRSA, go to your doctor for an evaluation of the inflammation or lesion. Practice extreme personal hygiene; do not use any personal items such as razors other than your own. Keep infected areas clean. A core prerequisite to good health lies in supporting and enhancing our immune system response. Boost your immune system with a natural immune boosting diet, rich in the colors yellow, orange, red and green. For extra support, look to supplements like astragalus, colostrum, zinc, vitamin C, vitamin A, beta-carotene, antioxidants and beta glucans found in medicinal mushroom such as agaricus blazei, reishi and maitake.

What is Colloidal Silver?

Colloidal silver is simply metallic silver suspended in water. A colloid describes microscopic particles suspended in a different material or environment. Silver boasts a stellar record in which not a single case of antibiotic resistant bacteria has surfaced, and works by smothering the bacterium.

Colloidal silver is not a newcomer in medical circles. Since ancient times, silver has been used as an antibiotic to treat a myriad of conditions. Colloidal silver works as a catalyst during the healing process as well as a disinfectant. It essentially suffocates the invaders by disabling the enzyme that bacteria and viruses require for the metabolism of oxygen.

Another way silver incapacitates disease causing organisms is through negative charges, which render the germs unable to reproduce. Along with taking silver internally, soak the affected area directly in the silver solution from fifteen minutes to an hour depending on the severity of the condition.

Dosage: Refer to manufacturer's recommendations. Sometimes it is suggested to take colloidal silver for three days and then stop for a few days (it usually takes three days for its effects to be felt). When consuming this product, swish it around in your mouth for 30 seconds before swallowing. This will give it a chance to absorb into the blood stream. You may also follow a professional health practitioner's recommendations depending on

---

the reason for taking the product, the dosage may vary. Most professional health food stores carry colloidal silver.

Silver Patches and Bandages: Clinical studies show that silver has powerful antibacterial agents that kill harmful germs, thus reducing the risk of infection. These unique pads within the bandage contain silver ions that are continually released during the healing process. Do not use ointments in combination with silver patches or bandages, as they will block the silver ions.

Turmeric: Turmeric has antibacterial properties and contains other medicinal elements that have been proven beneficial as a treatment for resistant bacterial strains. Simply observe a country known for having unsanitary living conditions, such as India, and yet which does not have superbugs running rampant. The reason is regular ingestion of turmeric. A United States study of 300 people who were all infected with MRSA showed very promising results; upon being surveyed, over 262 subjects said that they had completely recovered using a simple spice from the supermarket—turmeric.

Curcumin is the active constituent of turmeric indicated for *gastro-intestinal* complaints specifically, inflammatory conditions, loss of appetite, high cholesterol, heart support and many other body stressors.

Suggested dosage: 300 mg, or four capsules daily with meals

Garlic: To simply state that garlic and oil of oregano are versatile is a gross understatement. These herbs both have impressive healing profiles. A potent chemical called allicin, a compound extracted from garlic, has become a staple among health conscious people. Allicin not only holds an amazing track record at destroying even the most antibiotic-resistant strains of MRSA, but also new strains of bacteria that have developed resistance to the more powerful antibiotics, such as Vancomycin and Glycopeptides.

Suggested dosage: 1000–2000 mg, twice a day (and then a maintenance dosage)

Oil of Oregano: The naturally occurring compound carvocrol in oregano has been found to contain potent antibacterial and antifungal properties with a range of medicinal applications including wiping out MRSA and C-defficile. A research team at the University of West of England in Bristol found that even minute quantities of carvocrol is a more effective anti-microbial agent than the 18 pharmaceutical drugs it was compared to. The disinfectant agents within oregano are still viable even at boiling temperatures, which increases its usefulness in the areas of cleaning and laundry to prevent the spread of superbugs.

Suggested dosage: 4 drops mixed with water under the tongue 3 times a day, or as directed by product brand. Discontinue when healed.

Manuka Honey: The Manuka bush (*leptospermum scoparium*), the source of manuka honey, is native to New Zealand. Dr. Peter Molan MBE, Associate Professor in Biochemistry at the University of Waikato in New Zealand has shown that most honeys have varying degrees of healing properties due to a naturally occurring hydrogen peroxide agent. Dr. Molan and his research team have discovered that manuka honey possesses an extra antibacterial component not found in other honey. Manuka honey has been shown to be effective against MRSA strains of bacteria without harming our gut's good bacteria. Look for the UMF (unique manuka factor) when purchasing manuka honey, a measurement standard of the antibacterial potency within the honey (specifically, look for UMF 10+–16+.)

Suggested dosage: 2 teaspoons taken half an hour before a meal, 3 times a day.

Sutherlandia frutescens: The plant Sutherlandia is a well known medicinal herb, also called the cancer bush in South Africa. This herb's reputation for treating superbugs like MRSA or other resistant germs is earned due to its antiviral, anticancer and immune boosting qualities. A few of its main chemical components are L-Canavanine, Pinitol and GABA.

Suggested dosage: 300–600 mg, twice a day (morning and evening with a meal)

Probiotics: *Lactobacillus acidophilus* and *Bifidobacterium bifidum* have the unique ability to increase our body's built-in defense mechanisms. Probiotics assist in fighting superbugs and routinely balance certain pathogens in the body like H-pylori, yeast, fungus and e-coli to assist with the maintenance of normal intestinal health. Vancomycin and Teicoplanin are common drugs used to treat MRSA infections which upset the gastrointestinal tract. Probiotics help counter the uncomfortable side effects produced by the drugs. Refer to Chapter 9 for application and dosage information.

Other Suggestions: Tea tree oil and olive leaf extract are essential oils with similar capabilities to that of oregano oil, both of which have shown resistance to micro-organisms. Pau de'Arco is an herb found in Mexico that also kills viruses, fungi and bacteria. Finally, when contemplating a different approach, oxygen therapy is worth considering since MRSA and other bacterial strains have an aversion to oxygen.

In light of C-defficile, MRSA's and the ability of other superbugs to target the immune system so aggressively, even through the smallest break on the skin—any remedy should focus on disrupting these pathogens internally and externally.

CHAPTER EIGHT

Treat Depression and Stress Safely and Effectively with Non-Drug Remedies

The Stress Syndrome and Its Effects on Gut Diseases and the Body

Stress occurs at all levels in life. Traditionally, we've been taught to believe that "health" is merely "the absence of disease." It isn't until recently that the medical community has finally acknowledged that stress is not just in the mind, but in the body. Not only that, stress can actually be measured.

Controlling stress in your life is one of the most important measures in optimizing your health. Stress is an individual experience. How well we adapt to stress largely depends upon the health of our adrenal glands, the main component in surviving long periods of stress. Nutrient deficiencies can lead to physical and physiological stress, while inversely stress can deplete nutrients.

Today, strong evidence shows that a stressful lifestyle and increased exposure to environmental hazards are both directly linked to the following conditions, which have now become predictable occurrences among the general public: premature aging, heart disease, memory problems, obesity, hypertension, edema, hormone and sugar imbalances, impaired immune defense, and organ and glandular weaknesses.

The Role Stress Plays in Gastrointestinal Diseases
It has been said many times that stress does not cause Crohn's, colitis and celiac diseases (though irritable bowel syndrome is strongly linked to stress

and anxiety). As for inflammatory bowel disease (IBD), this has not been my complete experience; the cases have been few in numbers where life's stressful situations were the root cause that resulted in the patient acquiring the condition of Crohn's and colitis. More typically, I've noticed the affect that stress has upon the *symptoms* of inflammatory bowel disease. The root cause for a person's stress requires attention to restore balance and to minimize its impact. This can be anything from a minor annoyance to deep grief associated with death, or any other circumstances involving extreme heartache. Worry certainly tops the list, especially when a person cannot control their thoughts and it overrides everything else around them. A scenario such as this could lead to depression, another common condition associated with anyone dealing with a prolonged illness.

How Does Stress Affect Gut Disorders?
In cases where stress is not the direct cause, there is still an influence on the digestive tract. Stressful events trigger flare-ups involving diarrhea, nausea and inflammation. The stomach becomes more easily upset by the increased secretion of hydrochloric acid, brought on by unwanted thoughts and circumstances.

Causes of Stress in Gut Disorders
The mere thought of a possible flare-up while trying to maintain a normal daily routine is enough to trigger symptoms of irritable bowel syndrome (IBS) brought on by anxiety. As we have come to realize, stress is not going away. Managing a chronic illness is, in and of itself, a stressful situation. The many visits to the hospital and doctor's office, even just trying to find something to eat that won't trigger a reaction, is stressful. Stress management requires energy. Malabsorption brings on its own form of stress to the body. Lack of nutrition weakens the body lowering coping mechanisms, ultimately increasing stress levels.

Consequences of Acute and Chronic Stress
We don't all respond to stress in the same way; in fact, stress isn't always bad. But acute stress may be brief in duration, while being intense in symptoms. Chronic stress is defined as unresolved circumstances persisting over extended periods of time. The following is a brief look at how stress affects various parts and systems in the body.

Brain: *Acute stress* affects the brain by increasing alertness and decreasing the perception of pain. The effects of *chronic stress* on the brain can result in headaches, impaired memory, depression and disturbed sleep patterns. Prolonged stress also depletes certain neurotransmitters in the brain, which can trigger carbohydrate cravings and eating binges.

Adrenal glands: *Acute stress* overstimulates the adrenal glands by engaging in the "fight or flight" response. Normally, this would be fine if confronted by a predator; however, this response does not help if you're simply late for an appointment. *Chronic stress* raises cortisol levels, dampening responses to acute stress. High cortisol levels cause increased insulin release, weight gain, inflammation, and a chain reaction that impacts several other organs and systems; in particular, the thyroid and adrenal glands.

Immune system: The quick acting *acute response* of our natural immunity prompts the immune system to ready itself for infections from external sources such as bites, scrapes and punctures. *Chronic stress*, that which seems to be beyond a person's control or seems endless, results in suppressed functioning in almost all aspects of the immune system.

Reproductive organs: Sex and stress are physically entwined. *Acute stress* temporarily suppresses functioning in the reproductive system. The risk of miscarriage and increased infertility are associated with *chronic stress*. Elevated cortisol levels deplete the reserves of the hormone DHEA, involved in the production of sex hormones. Consequently, as sex hormones reduce, the libido begins to decline.

Circulatory system: Stress has a substantial affect on the circulatory system, which includes the heart, arteries and veins. *Acute stress* increases heart rate. *Chronic stress* affects the circulatory system by elevating blood pressure and blood flow to the muscles, putting one at risk of cardiovascular disease or stroke. Prolonged stress impedes the oxygenation process that is necessary to keep all the other organs, and the body as a whole, functioning normally.

Oxidative Stress: A normal byproduct of *acute and chronic stress*, oxidative stress is promoted by increased levels of cortisol. Cortisol has been dubbed the "age-accelerating hormone." It increases internal generations of free radicals, altering cells at a molecular level. Oxidative stress is a major factor in the following conditions: aging, Alzheimer's disease, arthritis, cancer, cardiovascular disease, depressed immune function, endocrine dysfunction, insulin resistance and diabetes, macular degeneration, neurological dysfunction/Parkinson's disease and obesity.

Key factors to ward off oxidative stress are a healthy diet and sufficient levels of antioxidant-protective nutrients. To achieve adequate protection, eat a plant rich diet and supplements including the following antioxidants: vitamins A, C and E, selenium, alpha lipoic acid, coenzyme Q10 and glutathione. Nutrients consumed in excess by the body when stressed include B5 (pantothenic acid), vitamin A, C and E, selenium, hydrochloric acid, iron, zinc, calcium and magnesium.

Stress Management through Diet and Supplements

Both acute and chronic stress generates copious amounts of free radicals from oxidative stress. Incorporating a diet rich in antioxidants will control oxygen damage and support you through the short-term stressful periods to avert the development of chronic stress.

Eating well and supplementing your diet with appropriate nutrients will enhance your coping skills. Unfortunately, during periods of high stress, most people's diets fall short. For this reason, supplementing with a high quality multi-vitamin and mineral formula with higher levels of natural carotenoids and antioxidants is essential.

Supplemental Protocol for Chronic Stress

The major groups of antioxidants comprise more than 600 carotenoids and more than 4000 polyphenols. *Carotenoids* are oil based. *Polyphenols* are water soluble.

Superoxide dismutase (SOD) is one of the body's built-in antioxidants, capable of destroying enormous amounts of free radicals. French researchers were successful in stabilizing SOD from deteriorating in the digestive tract, enabling absorption and availability to attack free radicals for extended periods of time. SOD hinders the succession of events that cause cells to age, which is associated with respiratory problems, memory loss, cardiovascular complaints, vision failure, joint degeneration and premature aging.

Suggested Dosage: 1000 mg, 1–2 times a day.

Alpha lipoic acid is considered one of the most unique antioxidants discovered, having the ability to target both water and fat-based tissues and organs. Being so incredibly versatile allows it to eradicate free radicals in any area of the body.

Suggested dosages vary from 100–500 mg, taken 2–3 times a day.

Dehydroepiandrosterone (DHEA) is the most abundant hormone in the body. It protects the body against stress by acting like a buffer, blocking corticosteroids, the stress hormones. Research shows that even young people experiencing chronic stress undergo severe drops in DHEA levels. Among the many conditions that DHEA can benefit include anti-aging, memory loss, menopause, andropause, fatigue, weight loss, enhanced immune system and cardiovascular support.

Suggested Dosage: First, perform a blood test to check DHEA levels in order to determine dosage. A common dosage for patients ages 50–60 is 50 mg, once a day.

Rhodiola rosea is known for increasing mental and physical stamina. In documented studies of work related stress, male and female physicians working night shifts experienced anti-fatigue benefits, a measurable increase in perceptive and cognitive cerebral functions, increased psychomotor function, and reduced mental fatigue when taking rhodiola rosea, as compared to the placebo group.

Suggested Dosage: 300 mg, taken 2–3 times a day.

5-Hydroxytryptophan (5-HTP) is reported to be one of the most naturally effective ways to control chronic psychological stress. This form of stress leads to depression, anxiety disorders and obesity. Stress in its many forms is implicated in a long list of chronic health problems.

Suggested Dosage: 500 mg, 1–3 times a day.

Ashwagandha is an herb of particular interest in combating stress, since it appears to block the breakdown of acetylcholine, a neurotransmitter involved in cognitive function and memory. In addition, it protects the brain during periods of increased oxidative stress.

Suggested Dosage: 500 mg, 1–2 times a day.

L-Theanine is an amino acid derived from green tea, useful for chronic stress and anxiety.

Suggested Dosage: 100 mg, 3–5 times a day (depending on stress levels).

B-vitamins, especially B6 or P5P (pyridoxal 5 phosphate) are key nutrients involved in healthy adrenal function and stress response.

Suggested Dosage: 100 mg, 1–2 times a day.

Magnesium and **calcium** are important anti-stress minerals. Stress hormones increase urinary excretion of magnesium, whereas calcium, under stressful situations, is quickly absorbed into the intestinal tract and excreted in the feces.

Suggested Dosage (Combination Formula): 1500 mg taken at bedtime. If taking magnesium alone for depression and stress: 300 mg, 3 times a day, with a small amount of protein (minerals require protein for absorption).

Stress and Time Management
The first and most important measure in stress management is developing a program whereby effective change can be made to either reduce or eliminate stress. By taking control of stressful situations, rather than being controlled by them, patients will start to create a lifestyle that better deals with stress. Remain realistic when scheduling the to-do list of your day. The two optimum times to start implementing change are first thing in the morning and in the evening. Start by getting up earlier to give yourself more time to prioritize your day, thus minimizing full-blown aggravations. This may involve shifting some work or children's activities. The second time is in the evening. All too often the family mealtime is compromised as you spend time shuttling children around or working too late.

   Exercise is an effective tool to burn off stress hormones and to divert your attention away from daily stressors. Moderate exercise, lasting twenty to thirty minutes, 3–4 times a week, can diminish mental and emotional stress.

   Relaxation is the opposite of stress. Allocate time for whatever mode of enjoyment you prefer. Choose from among the many relaxation techniques such as yoga, Tai chi, meditation, massage, gardening, reading, family pets and laughter.

   As you approach and comprehend the healing process, utilize safe and effective herbal remedies to assist in calming the external stressors of life, while relaxing the physical symptoms of your illness. Refer to "Drug-Free Ways to Aid Depression" later in this chapter for more calming solutions.

To take charge of your health, as your first line of defense, consider lifestyle factors and take appropriate dietary and supplemental action to reduce the inevitable health challenges linked with stress.

Drug Free Ways to Aid Depression and Anxiety

Mood disorders for all ages are bordering on epidemic proportions throughout the world. Our modern lifestyle has changed our inherent balance, primarily due to technology. We no longer rest when the sun goes down, or eat food that is whole and void of chemicals. Everywhere we look today, people are living at a high speed pace with little thought of their internal environment until they "crash." Most people run to their doctor demanding a quick fix. But drugs are no panacea.

Almost a third of patients do not respond to antidepressants, and the ones that do find the drugs less effective over time coupled by unpleasant side effects. A collective accumulation of internal and external problems can lead to a depressed state. It makes more sense to find natural, non-drug ways to correct the imbalance of neurotransmitters like serotonin and of other key elements involved with depression.

Depression and Gut Disorders
The frustrating dilemma for those who suffer with gut disorders is the awareness of a potential lifelong illness. Over time, this brings about feelings of depression. It isn't hard to visualize the fear surrounding social functions or activities. As depression progresses, so too will the person withdraw from life, becoming more isolated and unhappy. All people with gut disorders experience irritability, impatience and disappointment brought on by the feeling of limitation. Regardless of illness, the majority of people experience these same symptoms without the constant worry these afflicted individuals deal with on a daily basis.

Depression and IBS
The combined impact of depression and irritable bowel syndrome can wreak havoc on a person's attempts to control their symptoms. The threat of symptoms occurring induces anxiety, while any external anxiety

brings on IBS symptoms—a vicious cycle with no end in sight. Studies indicate that 60 percent of irritable bowel syndrome patients suffer from a psychological disorder like depression or anxiety. Since antidepressant drugs are frequently prescribed for these conditions, the following information will prove valuable for anyone coping with mood swings and sadness.

What Transmits Feelings of Depression

Symptoms of depression, including feelings of suicide, are usually brought on by reduced levels of neurotransmitters such as serotonin, norepinephrine and dopamine. Serotonin is a key buffer against depression. Similar to a speech defect that hinders communication, serotonin interferes with neurotransmitter activity, which may short circuit the brain's internal communication. Neurotransmitters regulate many of the body's activities, such as anger, joy, sleep, hunger, mobility and memory.

Depression May Be a Physical Cause

Depression may also be symptomatic of other medical conditions, such as hypothyroidism, anemia or diabetes. The thyroid is an emotional gland which forms a triad with the adrenals and pancreas, all interrelating, all with an effect on our mental state.

Thyroid

The symptoms of depression may be a sign that a person's thyroid is underactive. A low level of thyroid hormones can lead to feelings of despair and extreme sadness. The amino acid tyrosine is used by the body to make the neurotransmitter noradrenaline, which is found in lower levels in people who are depressed (it also boosts dopamine levels).

Anemia

Anemia can bring on feelings of depression by impairing iron absorption in the cells that regulate dopamine in the brain.

Diabetes

Recent research points to depression as a possible cause or trigger of diabetes. Studies show that people with diabetes have a greater risk of depression than people without this condition.

Folic Acid Alert

A clinical study performed at the Harvard Medical School by Dr. Fava, a director of the depression and research program, found that patients with low folate levels had a much lower response to antidepressants than those with normal levels.

Suggested dosage: 400 mcg (consider a blood test for exact requirement).

Rethink Your Diet

Our ancestor's diet consisted of mostly green plants and small animals, which were low in fat but high in cholesterol. As it turns out, low cholesterol levels do interfere with the regulation of serotonin. Since high levels of LDL would not be recommended, the suggestion would be to monitor both levels. Refer to Chapter 10 for more information on quality fats.

A question about carbohydrates springs to mind: carbohydrates *do* improve serotonin temporarily, but over the long run a high carb diet leaves you feeling low and sluggish. The diminishing sense of well-being partly stems from the elevated insulin levels, which in turn boosts the production of certain prostaglandins linked to depression.

Caution: Only carbs that are deemed safe are to be consumed. Individual eating regimes must be adhered to, according to each person's gut complaint.

Happy Foods

To help maintain healthy insulin and cholesterol levels, emphasize fruits, vegetables, whole grains and legumes while limiting sweets, processed and junk foods. At each meal, strive to consume a protein/fat/carbohydrate ratio of 30 percent/30 percent/40 percent. In addition, frequent small meals of 500 calories or less will keep insulin levels lower than large meals. A few suggestions of foods to help curb depression are omega 3 fatty acids rich foods, such as salmon, trout, walnuts, soybeans, and chocolate, which also boost levels of serotonin. Foods containing tryptophan, such as bananas, peanuts and turkey, produce a calming effect on the body.

For those individuals with specific diet plans, use only your allowed and recommended foods and beverages.

Exercise to Combat "The Blues"

A surprising study presented by the Society of Behavioral Medicine, conducted at the Duke Medical Centre, showed that even short workouts, as brief as eight minutes, were enough to enhance mood by reducing feelings of sadness, tension, fatigue, anger and confusion. Exercise is a natural serotonin booster (not to be linked with only joyful moods, but also with better overall health).

Drug and Herbal Interactions

In our recent history, there has been a lot of hype surrounding St. John's wort and certain other medications. I wish to provide clarity on what is taking place within the cells by way of drug and herbal interaction.

P-glycol protein is our cell's membrane pump. Properties in St. John's wort enhance this cellular pump. Think of people coming into a room and being ushered out the back door. What this relates to is that, for those who are taking medication for depression, the drug is designed to remain in the cell for a protracted period of time.

As a practitioner who works extensively with plant extracts, I do not see or experience the adverse interactions being shown in the literature today. This is mainly due to the fact that drugs are so overpowering and block sensory communication in the body. Plants, in their whole, unadulterated state do not possess overwhelming isolated compounds that would be similar in nature to a drug's action. There are known interactions, like grapefruit extract and some vitamin and mineral absorption inhibitors, but in the larger picture any of these contraindications pale in comparison to how medications interfere with the protein pathways in the body. Drugs do not follow the holistic pathway in the body, and thereby interfere with all body functions.

This is just one reason why people feel worse when the prescriptions start to pile up. Even if you were to take St. John's wort with a drug that is performing the same task and is fractionally lessening the efficacy of the drug, the effects upon the body are far greater from the drug compared to the effects of the herb upon the drug.

Now, an area where one *does* want the drug to hang about the cells is in immune suppressant medications, such as those used in organ transplants. Patients of this nature are entrenched in traditional medicine. Professionals like myself rarely if ever see these types of patients. It's not that we *can't* help them, especially in assisting them with the toxic side effects from their medications. This is problematic, since these drugs wear out the kidneys (along with other severe complications).

Most, if not all drug and herbal interactions are theory-based. The trials and studies are not taking place. It's not that they shouldn't be, but the variables extant amongst the research subjects present a problem. The studies taking place are typically too small, and the symptoms, medications (including dosages) and plant chemistry need to be the same for accuracy—something that is very hard to come by. Research is looking at related compounds in each, assuming that there could be an adverse reaction. For example, if a drug is metabolized by caffeine and there is caffeine in the herb, they automatically assume that there is going to be an interaction.

My aim is to ignite your curiosity into doing your own investigative work by seeking the full studies many statements are taken from. I encourage my readers to form their own opinions and broaden their knowledge base for future decision making.

Non-Drug Alternatives to Treat Depression

Tryptophan: Tryptophan is an amino acid, available in a dietary supplement form as tryptophan or 5-HTP. Tryptophan is converted by the body into 5-hydroxytryptophan and then into serotonin.

Suggested Dosage: 500 mg, 1–3 times a day.

St. John's Wort: The herb St. John's wort has traditionally been used to treat all forms of nerve and emotional disorders. Herbs are often preferred over antidepressants due to having far fewer side effects.

Suggested Dosage: 10–15 drops of extract 3–6 times a day (or as needed).

SAM-e: SAM-e is a naturally occurring molecule that is involved in a number of metabolic functions, including the neurotransmitters serotonin and dopamine that are imbalanced in people who suffer with depression.

Suggested Dosage: 400 mg, 2–4 times a day.

Glutamine: Glutamine is an amino acid used by the body to make the neurotransmitter glutamate. Glutamate is promoted as a "brain food," inducing more energy and improving mood.

Suggested Dosage: 500 mg, 1–3 times a day.

Phenylalanine: Phenylalanine is an amino acid used by the body to make the neurotransmitter norepinephrine. The goal in supplementing phenylalanine is to prompt the brain to yield more norepinephrine.

Suggested Dosage: 1000 mg, 1–3 times a day.

Inositol: Inositol is a type of sugar related to glucose. Since low levels of inositol have been found in the spinal fluid of people with depression and in the brains of those who have committed suicide, inositol is being promoted as a useful treatment for mood disorders.

Suggested Dosage: Most brands are in a powder form, of which ¼ teaspoon is equivalent to 730–750 mg. Depending on the severity of the condition, take ¼–½ teaspoon three times a day.

Passionflower: Passionflower is primarily used for its sedative effects and for relieving gastrointestinal complaints. (Refer to "Discover Passionflower's Calming and Healing Benefits" in this chapter for additional information and dosages).

Tyrosine: Tyrosine is an amino acid used by the body to manufacture noradrenaline, which has shown to be in short supply in the brains of people with mood disorders.

Suggested Dosage: 500 mg, 1–3 times a day.

Other Suggestions: Complementary treatments for depression are wide and varied. Other suggestions include: light therapy, negative air ionization, music, yoga, meditation, vitamin/minerals, melatonin, homeopathy and herbal remedies.

The treatment of inflammatory bowel diseases (IBD) is particularly challenging because of their unpredictability. The atmosphere of helplessness and confusion accompanies Crohn's, colitis, celiac and irritable bowel syndrome. Feelings of despair always loom when there is a threat of symptoms flaring up. Life becomes extremely stressful. Depression is looked upon as one of the worst illnesses of our modern day society. To take claim of your mental health, consider lifestyle factors while incorporating a dietary and supplemental regime to reduce the unavoidable mood swings and health challenges associated with depression.

Discover Passionflower's Calming and Healing Benefits

Passionflower is one of the most researched herbs in existence, with a long history in traditional medicine. In recent times, it has even been integrated into clinical procedures.

Living in a time where anxiety is a constant companion to so many, passionflower has found its place as a healing agent, helping to re-establish inner harmony.

About Passionflower

Passionflower is indigenous to South and North America, favoring tropical areas. There are over 500 species of this woody vine, which bears impressive large white flowers with a pink and purple center. The parts used in herbal medicine include the vine, leaves and stem. Passionflower has traditionally been used as a sedative and for relief of gastrointestinal complaints. Currently, its therapeutic use has reached into the following areas: congestive heart failure, anxiety, asthma, insomnia, seizures, hysteria, ADHD, alcohol and drug withdrawal, antibacterial agent, infections, chronic pain, high blood pressure, menopausal symptoms and cancer. The list for application extends much further.

Today, passionflower is primarily used for its sedative and anxiety relieving effects, either as a single herb preparation or in combination with other plant extracts. Passionflower has been measured against such drugs as Diazepam (valium), Oxazepam, Lorazepam (Ativan), and Mexazolam, displaying equal anxiolytic benefits.

Active Plant Constituents

The active components found within passionflower are comprised mainly of three groups of chemicals: alkaloids, glycosides and flavonoids. Other key elements include the presence of antibacterial compounds, passicol and cyanogenic glycosides. Harmane indole alkaloids are another key feature of passionflower. Through scientific research, this group of alkaloids has demonstrated antispasmodic activity and the ability to lower blood pressure. The flavonoids portion in this species is estimated at 3 percent. *Passiflora incarnate* has been found to contain the highest concentration of these active properties by comparison. Naturally occurring serotonin and the chemical maltol are present in passionflower, which have documented sedative and calming effects.

Research also supports the enhancing effects of passionflower when combined with other plant extracts such as St. John's wort. On a different note, Perry, et al (1991) indicated *Passiflora tetrandra*'s potential as a plant derived antibiotic. New strategies and alternative approaches have become necessary to destroy and prevent recurring infections from superbugs and staph bacterium.

Evidence for Medicinal Indications

- Anxiety Relief: A well-known double blind study published in the *Journal of Clinical of Pharmacy and Therapeutics* took place over a four week period where individuals suffering from anxiety attacks were intensely scrutinized. The comparison of passionflower to the commonly prescribed drug Oxazepam, showed the extract of passionflower to be equally effective by the end of the four week period. Passionflower showed lesser side effects overall, including daytime and job restrictions, as compared to Oxazepam.
- ADHD: A comparative study involving children diagnosed with ADHD examined the effects of passionflower to the commonly prescribed stimulant drugs over an eight week period. The outcome showed similar effectiveness in treating ADHD, with fewer side effects, in the passionflower group.
- Congestive Heart Failure: A collaborative study by Eiff, Brunner and Haegeli showed improvement in physical exercise capacity of patients with dysponea (difficult breathing) using a hawthorn/passionflower extract. Since it is often difficult to have enough scientific evidential studies conducted in the arena of natural medicine, further study is recommended for congestive heart failure.
- Anti-Microbial Activity: Passicol is an antibacterial and antifungal agent produced by the Passiflora plant species. Researchers such as Britto (2001), Afolayan and Meyer (1997) and Balakrishna (2000) all confirmed that the plant's extracts exhibited anti-bacterial activity when tested against known pathogenic bacterial strains such as Streptococcus, V. cholerae, Bacillus cereus, Escherichia coli, Pseudomonas putida and aeruginosa, Shigella flexneri, fungus and yeasts.

- Drug Addiction: A 14-day, double blind study of 65 men afflicted with opiate (heroin) addiction compared the effectiveness of passionflower in combination with and as a stand alone remedy to a drug routinely used to assist narcotic withdrawal, Clonidine. Clonidine is effective at reducing physical symptoms, such as high blood pressure, but has no effect on the patient's emotional symptoms such as nervousness, anxiety, depression and chemical cravings.
  - Passionflower, when partnered with Clonidine, was successful by a significant margin at relieving the emotional aspects of withdrawal symptoms as compared to the drug alone. These findings were particularly important, since it is the emotional symptoms which often halt the progress of individuals trying to complete their drug treatment program.
- Pre-Surgery Anxiety: Passiflora incarnate significantly reduced anxiety when administered to 60 patients ninety minutes prior to surgery in a placebo controlled trial, supervised by Movafegh, A. et al. (2008).
- Other Uses: Passionflower is a well-researched herb, as indicated by Germany's rigorous Commission E approving its use for nervous restlessness and by the British Herbal Compendium approving the use of passionflower for restlessness, sleep disorders, nervous stress and anxiety.

Dosages
The following dosage recommendations are only a general guideline. The amounts may vary according to brands and when administered by a qualified practitioner.

Safety: Passionflower is on the FDA's GRAS (Generally Recognized as Safe) list.

Adults (18 years or older): Dried herb: 0.5 grams (.5 ml/1/8 tsp) taken 3–4 times per day. Alternative: 2–3 grams in tablets or capsules, taken 2–3 times per day.

Tincture: 1–4 milliliters (1:8) or 20–80 drops taken 3–4 times per day on the tongue or in liquid.

Tea: 4–8 grams (1–2 teaspoons) of dried herb steeped in one cup of water, 1–3 times per day.

Pediatric Dosage: A child's weight is taken into account when adjusting the recommended adult dose. A typical herbal dosage for adults is intended for an adult's weight of 150 pounds. If the weight of the child is 50 pounds, the appropriate amount of passionflower for this child would be 1/3 of the adult dose. Refer to Chapter 11 to determine children's dosages.

Drug Interactions and Contraindications: None reported.

In theory, sedative effects may be possible when coupled with sedative drugs and other plant extractions of the same nature.

For most of us, living a life of tranquility without any stressors happens only when we are day-dreaming. Regardless of the form in which stress appears, sometimes the body's coping mechanisms cannot sustain a healthy balance. Left unchecked, the entire body becomes affected. During such times, the body initiates a constant state of readiness, which often leads to exhaustion. As we seek out help, a step toward serenity just may be in the form of a woody vine bearing unusually striking flowers called "passionflower."

CHAPTER NINE

Best Immune and Healing Support

What is Colostrum?

Colostrum is an amazing substance that is produced in nature by mothers for their newborns, and which is instrumental in nourishing the child's immune system. Colostrum is often referred to as "the first mother's milk before real milk comes." Biologically, colostrum has more protein and fat than the normal milk produced by mothers and contains antibodies which protect the newborn against illness.

Colostrum Empowers the Body to Heal

Colostrum is one of those overlooked miracles which has—up until now—been kept hush-hush. There have been over ten thousand clinical studies regarding colostrum, all published in peer reviewed journals, and yet not one of these amazing findings ever made their way into publication where they could be accessed by the general public. Luckily, the nutraceutical industry has recently begun embracing this substance, in turn opening the door to its amazing health-promoting properties. Colostrum benefits any disorder that requires extra attention from the immune system. As such, this complex healer is a must-have for people who suffer from gastrointestinal disorders.

When you are researching colostrum, like any other substance or foods, also research its components or elements and their properties, not just the name of the item itself.

> TIP: For example, if you were to research any other wonderful health food, such as the Acai berry, and how it may help cancer or diabetes, you will get much further if you look up the properties in the berries that are actually being used in studies (in this case, anthocyanins in the Acai berry, and cancer or diabetes).

Properties and Benefits of Colostrum

At present, colostrum is under appreciated and underutilized by the health industry. Let's take a brief look at some of the many benefits that colostrum has to offer. More awareness may be needed to help conventional medicine start recommending this product more often.

Colostrum Benefits Include Chronic Gut Disorders

Colostrum provides a perfect combination of amino acids, immune growth factors (such as immunoglobulin, lactoferrin, and insulin-like growth factor also referred to as 1 (IGF)) and other immune boosting properties.

A long list of studies and trials in the field of all forms of inflammatory bowel diseases, irritable bowel syndrome and celiac, report patients feeling better with reduced symptoms upon taking colostrum. These reduced and improved symptoms include: less bleeding, reduced gastrointestinal irritation, quicker healing and repair of damaged intestinal tissue, especially from the use of NSAIDs like Motrin, Advil, or Ibuprofen.

Dosage suggestion: 500 mg, twice a day.

> Several years ago, Doug Wyatt's wife Kaye needed colostrum, because her thymus had been destroyed by radiation treatments. Fortunately, and through due diligence, Doug spent time, money and tremendous effort to expose the benefits of colostrum and bring it to America. Kaye had to have a bit of colostrum every day for immune protection. In a case such as her's, when adequate protection is not provided from the immune glands, even a cold could end your life.
>
> What Doug discovered was that high-quality colostrum was only available in New Zealand. He and his company, called Symbiotics, collaborated with the New Zealand government and reached an agreement to sell colostrum in the United States and further distribute the product throughout the world.

Colostrum's Effects on Immune Deficient Patients
There are several scientific studies supporting and demonstrating the protective effects of colostrum. One such study involved an influenza trial that resulted in three times more benefit compared to vaccinations. Because of its natural defense arsenal, colostrum's beneficial properties also include anti-bacterial, anti-fungal, anti-viral, anti-parasitic, and anti-tumoral activities. Lactoferrin, another component of colostrum, promotes bone growth and enhances the recovery of the immune system. A few other benefits to patients include dental health, diabetics, allergies, wound healing and protection to the intestinal epithelium.

Note: When purchasing colostrum, inquire as to its packaging and preparation. The quality of the product, as with all other natural products, is of utmost importance.

Colostrum Sources: Nature's Harmony, Symbiotics, Now Foods, Vitamin Shoppe, ChildLife Gold, and California Gold Nutrition.

Probiotics Benefits Crohn's Disease and All Other Gastrointestinal Complaints

Probiotics has become the casual term for the microflora *Lactobacillus acidophilus* and *Bifidobacterium bifidum*, both of which support the body by balancing other threatening pathogens; they are even utilized by the thyroid gland, as will be discussed later on. Probiotics play an intricate role in our internal biology. It has even been said that, unless one balances one's own internal microbial or microflora, conditions such as Crohn's, ulcerative colitis, celiac and irritable bowel syndrome can never be fully reversed. As a practitioner who deals with many gastrointestinal disturbances, this area of health is always part of my therapeutic programming. Even with constipation, the imbalance of e-coli, lactobacillus and bifidus within the large colon has an impact on the transit time of bowel movements, as well as the color and texture of the fecal matter itself.

About Probiotics
Friendly flora is another accepted name for various strains of beneficial bacteria. The FAO/WHO describes probiotics as, "Live microorganisms which, when administered in adequate amounts, confer a health benefit on the host." This type of bacterial flora is not new, occurring naturally

in many different fermented foods which have been consumed by various cultures for centuries. Over a hundred years ago, a Russian biologist named Elie Metchnikoff, best remembered for his pioneering research into the immune system, received the Nobel Prize in Medicine in 1908. He is also known for his study of aging and longevity. It was when working in the area of fermented foods that he noticed people who ate these foods lived longer and were healthier.

Probiotics play an important part in our overall immunity. Many people do not realize that our internal environment must be balanced, especially in terms of pathogens. What's more, the general public is unaware of their involvement in their body's functions. Imagine that you are now eating a really healthy diet but you have no awareness of what *else* is feeding off the food you have just eaten. Food is the energy source for the body's multitude of tasks. Once food has been broken down into minute particles, it becomes a food source for the various life forms inhabiting the body.

Probiotics Perform Major Tasks
- 20 percent of thyroid gland functions *depend* on probiotics— our friendly flora.
- The stomach is a vital area requiring these friendly microbes to keep *H. pylori* in balance, a bacterium which often precipitates a stomach ulcer.
- Fungus and candida are kept in check by probiotics, as is e-coli in the large colon.
- Other than the thyroid gland and stomach, lactobacillus acidophilus occupy the small intestine and large colon.
- Probiotics is one way to keep pathogens at bay; after all, these life forms are gobbling up the nutrients that are meant to feed your blood and tissues.
- Common yeast infections (candidiasis) and childhood related ailments such as cradle cap and diaper rash are related to insufficient amount of probiotics and too much sugar in the diet. Even bipolar disorder may be the outcome of too much fungus building up in the brain.

Antibiotic Associated Diarrhea
The use of probiotics in the prevention and treatment of antibiotic associated diarrhea has improved conditions of Crohn's disease and all other

gut disorders. Research has left no doubt as to the significant benefits of probiotics, warranting their application as a treatment for gastrointestinal disturbances. Probiotics have also been shown to improve lactose intolerance implicated in Crohn's, ulcerative colitis and celiac diseases.

Crohn's Disease Trouble Spots

Research reveals that we have *hundreds* of different micro-bacteria species occupying our colon (although there are far fewer numbers living in the stomach and small intestine, compared to the large colon). One of the reasons we find less bacterial invasion in the stomach and upper intestine is due to our stomach's hydrochloric acid, which produces a highly acidic environment promoting unsuitable surroundings for bacterial survival. Because of the differentiating areas of bacteria population, the area near the bottom of the small intestine joining the large colon is a targeted area call the ileum.

There are several symptomatic steps involving the onslaught of Crohn's disease which can be both fairly general among patients or an uncommon individual incidence. What *is* common among patients is the unwanted microbes that over proliferate and seep into the small intestine.

Probiotics are one of the tools used to protect against the overabundance of harmful microbial species within the gut system. Once the equilibrium of the colon is imbalanced, a series of occurrences start to play out, such as an overloading of the gut with waste by-products from microbes, an overburdening of the immune system, an impairment of vitamin B absorption and nutrition malabsorption, which is then followed by physical symptoms.

Probiotics continue to be recommended for their diverse applications in alleviating gastrointestinal complaints from *H. pylori* to infections and colon cancer. Consequently, in outlining treatment therapies for an individual, programs should always include appropriate dosages of probiotics.

Monitoring Candida Benefits All Gut Disorders

Candidiasis is considered to be a twentieth century disease. Yeast infections most frequently strike women, prompted by a yeast-type fungus named candida, which normally populates the intestinal tract. A weakened immune system, certain medications, allergies, hormonal changes, high sugar intake and a poor diet are usually the main causes of yeast infections.

The single greatest cause of yeast overgrowth is the overuse of antibiotics. Since antibiotics are routinely given for gut dysbiosis problems and kill randomly, an imbalance between the good intestinal flora and the bad is created. To prevent recurring bouts of candida, the diet must be addressed to promote health and an adverse environment for yeast to proliferate.

Lactobacillus acidophilus and bifidobacterium bifidum are beneficial bacteria that strive to balance our internal environment. These friendly bacteria are known for combating candida overgrowth, neutralizing pathogens such as e-coli and salmonella while fighting infection. Probiotics come in live culture or freeze dried capsule form, as well as in cultured dairy products like kefir and plain yogurt. For those who are allergic to dairy, non-dairy products can be purchased. Suggested dosage (total bacterial culture): 10 billion bacterium per capsule, 1–3 times a day.

To control candida, eliminate sugar in all its various forms from the diet, as candida thrives on sugar. Avoid sweet fruit, processed foods like ketchup and white flour products. Restrict alcohol, as it may be composed of fermented and refined sugar.

For aggressive elimination of candida, various supplements have proven beneficial. Caprylic acid is a plant substance with naturally occurring antifungal properties, compared to the prescription drug nystatin. Likewise, citrus seed extracts and garlic are effective. Suggested dosage for caprylic acid is to take twice a day for 3–4 weeks with a meal. Follow manufacturer's recommended amounts and take as directed.

All EFAs (essential fatty acids) have strong antifungal properties. Fish oil and flax seed oil are excellent sources of omega 3 fatty acids. Evening primrose oil, borage, wheat germ and black currant oils are high in omega 6 fatty acids. Niacin and biotin are B vitamins; along with vitamin C, which possesses antifungal action. Consume lots of fresh, raw vegetables and juices, non-sweet fruits, mineral water and herbal teas to eliminate toxins. Green food supplements, with their high chlorophyll content, strengthen the immune system while inhibiting candida overgrowth. Prior to antifungal medications, iodine found in kelp and dulse was the main treatment for fungus and candida.

Herbal remedies such as calendula, horsetail, aloe vera, ginger, goldenseal and echinacea have the capacity to eliminate and control the growth of harmful bacteria, along with the ability to soothe and repair intestinal tissue.

Treatment of candida for infants and children consists of changing to a high fiber diet (child appropriate) and natural remedies, to include probiotics. Green food supplements such as chlorophyll or barley greens will boost their immune system. Apply topical creams containing zinc, calendula and aloe vera to affected areas requiring healing. Be aware that the problem often stems from the high sugar content found in commercial baby foods, juices and dairy products.

Carrot Juice Quickens the Healing Process of Crohn's Disease and All Other Gut Abnormalities

Diseases such as Crohn's, as well as most other gastrointestinal complaints, have several commonalities in the area of food intolerances. Patients in acute stages find it difficult to digest many substances, and malnourishment is always a complication. Part of my initial protocol in treating these ailments always involves the juicing of carrots as a primary ingredient.

Unadulterated raw food in the form of easily assimilated carrot juice is highly beneficial for Crohn's patients and other gastrointestinal disorders. The benefits range from its nutritional value, to boosting and supporting the immune system and accelerating the healing processes, along with other major functions and systems throughout the body.

The availability of nutrients utilized in this form of nutrition is unbeatable. Think of the fine, delicate root fibers of a carrot; once the minerals past through this intricate maze, the job is complete. The body does not need to break down any mineral compounds in order to digest this fluid.

Nutritional Benefits
Carrot juice is teeming with immune supporting nutrients which are invaluable to a patient with Crohn's, or other similar ailments. Elements such as falcarinol and beta carotene found in carrot juice are ideal for enhancing restoration of gut tissue, and healing lesions and broken capillaries.

Liquid vs. Whole Food
Plant fiber is often a problem for anyone suffering from gut complaints, especially in the initial stages of healing. Carrot juice provides nutritional value without the difficulty of assimilation and irritation of the digestive tract that can be seen with fiber.

Diarrhea is a Major Concern with Gut Disorders
At the University of Maryland's Medical Center, Steven D. Erlich, N.MD, recommended carrot for the treatment of diarrhea, a common complaint of patients with gastrointestinal disorders. Loss of electrolytes and other elements is a constant problem for anyone experiencing frequent diarrhea. Carrot juice is wonderful for returning the balance of these lost nutrients and fluids.

Nutritional Value of Consuming Carrot Juice
Individuals with Crohn's and other gastrointestinal problems typically have difficulty ingesting or retaining the nutritional properties of food. Carrot juice supplies a wide variety of vitamins and minerals, providing valuable nourishment to the patient while assisting the healing process. Studies indicate that regular ingestion of falcarinol reduces one's cancer risk by up to 40 percent.

Falcarinol is Protective to Plants and People
Falcarinol is a relative newcomer, but is now topping the list of elements that have a profound impact on our health. This property found in carrots serves as the plant's natural pesticide and an antioxidant to consumers. Dr. Kirsten Brandt, head of the research department at Newcastle University, explains, "Isolated cancer cells grow more slowly when exposed to falcarinol." For retaining the maximum amount of falcarinol, preparation is key. During the cooking process, carrots should not be sliced—cook them whole to retain their anti-cancer properties. Juicing is also highly recommended.

Beta-Carotene
Beta-carotene is synonymous with carrots. Other good sources are pumpkin, sweet potato, apricot, sweet peppers and greens. Beta-carotene is an antioxidant and a pre-cursor used to make vitamin A. This potent compound is well recognized for enhancing many immune system processes and has been noted to help reduce a wide range of cancers.

Other Common Deficiencies Related to Gut Dysbiosis

Carrot juice supports nutrient deficiencies in gut-related complaints, including zinc, folic acid, calcium and vitamins A, D, and K. Carrot juice is also a fine source of B vitamins, in addition to vitamins C and E. Calcium is known as the "knitter" in the body, helping to repair the intestinal walls. Zinc and vitamin A really boost the immune system. Other aspects of healing are the antioxidants in fresh raw juices, which assist in reducing pain while strengthening tissue such as the delicate capillaries (which promote bleeding when they rupture). These valuable components are lost to heat and processing.

As a practitioner, I have noticed that when a patient incorporates the juicing of vegetables with carrots as the primary ingredient, they experience an increase in energy and an enhancement to their healing process. I always promote raw vegetable juicing where healing and restoration of tissue is required. In the case of gastrointestinal disorders, depending on the condition and the initial stage of complications, I recommend consuming anywhere from one pint (500 ml or ½ liter) once a day to one pint three times a day for quicker healing results. Other vegetables may be added to the formula depending on individual requirements. Juicing carrots with beet root and greens is one of my favorite tools to boost vitality and the overall health of my patients.

Aloe Vera Promotes Healing of Crohn's Disease, Ulcerative Colitis, Celiac, IBS and Other Gastrointestinal Complaints

Crohn's sufferers have a long list of concerns and complaints. Disorders such as Crohn's and colitis are commonly associated with symptoms of pain, inflammation, gas, bloating, bleeding, diarrhea, indigestion, constipation, abscesses and fistulas. It has been my experience that most people are initially looking to alleviate symptoms of discomfort which prompts the question, "What will heal me and take away my discomfort?" Amongst the top healing plants, aloe vera holds a high ranking position. Aloe vera has earned its reputation as a great healing agent, and has been used internally and externally for centuries.

What is Aloe Vera?
Aloe vera is a succulent plant with thick fleshy green leaves. As far back as the first century C.E., aloe vera was used medicinally as it continues to be today. As a species, many feel it originated in northern Africa. Its extracts are used internally and externally with a wide range of benefits. Aloe vera

contains a vast array of nutrients, numbering 200 or more. Within this remarkable plant are vitamins, minerals, amino acids, antioxidants and enzymes. These nutrients form the base for good health and are easily assimilated by the body.

The reason for this is that this versatile plant possesses long chain polysaccharides that repair the tiny holes within the gut. Throughout the healing process, aloe vera reduces inflammation, pain and bleeding—all of which are primary symptoms causing distress and discomfort.

One of the physical attributes of Crohn's disease and other gut complaints is leaky gut syndrome and permeable tissue lining. As a result of these holes in the gut, unwanted particles pass through into the blood. For example, substances such as gluten protein, once in the blood, signal the immune system to attack and destroy. If this occurrence is repeated continually, the offending protein becomes a trigger, recognized by the immune system as a foreign and harmful element. The gut lining must be healed over to prevent leakage of foreign material which could otherwise initiate this immune response. Even when the intestinal tract has had sufficient time to heal, other influences can still trigger an immune response (refer to Chapter 12 for more information on the brain connection).

Resolving leaky gut syndrome is initially a two step process. First, the substances which trigger the immune response must be removed until such time as the body has healed and no longer recognizes the substance as harmful. Secondly, during this elimination process, the gut can commence the reversal process, promoting tissue integrity once again. This is accomplished by additionally supporting the immune system and the body with healing and health promoting substances like aloe vera.

Fortunately, the cells in our intestinal tract replicate very quickly, and are replaced approximately every four days. Aloe, containing nutrients such as the amino acid L-glutamine (which is in great demand by these cells) enhances the restoration of intestinal tissue. As I tell my patients time and again, nature has the remedy to aid our needs, waiting to be called upon so that it may have the opportunity to work synergistically with our bodies.

CHAPTER TEN

Necessary Elements for a Disease Reversal Process

Omega 3 Fatty Acids (EFAs) are Essential for Rebuilding Tissue and Improving Longevity

Today's scientific research has enlightened us on the subject of healthy fats. Yet these explorative studies have shown that most of the general public does not consume the proper amount of omega 3 fatty acids; the average intake is nowhere near the proportion necessary to support and regenerate the body. This inadequate amount of beneficial fats (omega 3 fatty acids), coupled with high levels of less desirable fats, creates an imbalance that leads to deficiencies in required fats. In this chapter, we'll be discussing what the body needs on a daily basis, the correct ratio of necessary nutrients, and how to go about balancing your diet to ensure adequate consumption of these essential nutrients.

To start with, we consume an excess of omega 6 fatty acids (grain and vegetable oil). This ratio should be 1:1 (1 portion omega 6 EFAs to 1 portion omega 3 EFAs). To better illustrate the importance of this information, I have included examples of essential areas and major systems within the body which require omega 3 fatty acids in order to perform their functions and rebuild tissue. Additionally, there is a significant difference in these fatty acids in terms of how and where they are used, as well as in their structure.

EPA/DHA Fatty Acids

Essential fatty acids, especially from coldwater fish, are abundant with EPA (eicosapentaenoic acid) and DHA (docosahexaenoic acid). Omega 3 fatty acids are referred to as EFAs (essential fatty acids) or PUFAs (polyunsatu-rated fatty acids). These fats require their correct balance in order to be uti-lized throughout the body. Dietary sources of omega 3 fatty acids include fish oils and seed oils such as flax seed oil, hemp oil, chia oil and walnut oil.

What is the Difference Between Fish Oil and Seed Oil?
- Fish oil differs from plant-based oils in that fish oil has long chained fatty acids, while seed oils have short chained fatty acids.
- Only long chained omega 3 fatty acids have the ability to feed the brain and the body, whereas plant omega 3s nourish other parts of the body

Do Vegetarians and Vegans Get Enough Long Chain Fatty Acids?
An article was published in the American Journal of Clinical Nutrition (2010) in which it was concluded that the conversion rate from plant based alpha-linolenic acid (ALA) intake to long chain EPA and DHA is actually increased (or made more efficient) in vegetarians and vegans. The concern lies in whether or not vegetarian and vegans are getting enough long chain fatty acids, as these fats are primarily found in fish (and some algae). The conversion rate from short chain fatty acids to long chain is slow and incomplete.

The suggestion for remedying this problem was to take a 1:1 ratio of omega 6 and omega 3 plant-based fatty acids. To achieve this ratio, extra attention must be paid to consuming sufficient ALA to ensure the preser-vation of adequate DHA levels. To protect against an imbalance, the ratio works out to be 4:1, or 4 parts omega 3s (such as flax and chia oil) to 1 part omega 6 fatty acids (found in olive and vegetable oils and certain amounts in seed and nut oils).[7]

What Are Some of the Major Areas Requiring Omega 3 Fatty Acids?
- Our brain mass consists of 60 percent or more of omega 3 fatty acids. By regularly ingesting long chain fatty acids such as fish oil or krill, this brain mass is enhanced. Additionally, consuming these long chain fatty acids protects the brain mass

---

7   Reference: Harnack K, Andersen G, Somoza V. Quantitation of alpha-linolenic acid elongation to eicosapentaenoic and docosahexaenoic acid as affected by the ratio of n6/n3 fatty acids. Nutr Metab (Lond). 2009; 6:8.

you currently have against shrinkage and conditions leading to Alzheimer's disease.

- Almost every brain disorder benefits from optimal levels of omega 3 fatty acids (EPA and DHA fatty acids).
- Nerve communication cannot occur in a normal way without omega 3 fatty acids. Omega 3 fatty acids are critical to the structure and function of neuronal membranes, in that they assist in transmitting information by electrical and chemical signaling. Omega 3 fatty acids are a core component of the nervous system, including the brain spinal cord, sensory glands and like.
- Omega 3 fatty acids aid cholesterol balancing in the liver. The liver needs the right kind of fat in order to make cholesterol, and is a necessary component of the glands making hormones.
- Omega 3 fatty acids are required elements in manufacturing cell membranes (cellular walls). Remember, we have 5 *trillion* cells in our bodies.
- Omega 3 fatty acids help in controlling inflammation responses, which lead to pain and the spread of disease. EPA and DHA essential fats are converted into active, hormone-like chemicals called prostaglandins. Prostaglandins have very strong anti-inflammatory properties.
- Omega 3 helps in initiating immune response, which requires an omega 3 fatty acid.
- Omega 3 controls hormone production.
- Omega 3 preserves the blood level of vitamin D.
- Baby aspirin (used for thinning the blood) can be replaced with adequate amounts of EPA s and DHAs, such as found in omega 3 fatty acids.
- Nattokinase may be considered if you are on blood thinners and wish to investigate reducing or stopping this form of medication. Seek professional counseling in monitoring any change. Serrapeptase and proteinase are two other protcolytic enzymes with greater potency that increase circulation. Product quality is critical.
- ADHD is benefited by omega 3, as EFAs are needed for proper retinal and brain development.

Dr. Harris W.C. and colleges performed 25 clinical trials on post heart attack patients who consumed as little as 850 mg per day of fish oil.

Remarkably, the outcome showed a 30 percent reduction in cardio vascular mortality and 45 percent reduction in sudden cardiac death. All of these heart studies showed the benefit of omega 3 EFAs in preventing the blood from becoming too "sticky" and forming arterial blockages. Doctors recommend 1000 mg per day of fish oil for this condition.

An inflammation study investigating the interactions between an inflammatory molecule (Leukotrienes), fish oil and olive oil found that fish oil reduced inflammation by 30 percent, whereas subjects given olive oil were unchanged. For treating chronic pain and inflammation, a dosage of 4000–8000 IU in divided doses taken throughout the day with food is very helpful. Another study investigated the influence of fish oil and diet on the intestinal tissues of ulcerative colitis, Crohn's and control patients. The most noticeable anti-inflammatory effects were seen in the tissues of the ulcerative colitis patient. Fish oil as well is very beneficial for rheumatoid arthritis and other joint pain where swelling is involved.

Studies have also shown that the following conditions have all been linked to a deficiency of omega 3 fatty acids: heart health issues, Alzheimer's, dementia, allergies, depression, high blood pressure, asthma, eczema, learning disabilities, gut disorders and constipation.

Ratio: How to Balance these Fats on a Daily Basis.
While the correct ratio is 1:1—one part omega 6 fatty acids to one part omega 3 fatty acids, the average North American diet consists of ratios closer to 20:1 or 30:1. Most of the population has been consuming too many omega 6 fatty acids, so diet adjustments should concentrate on omega 3s. The body requires a great deal more omega 3s to regenerate and function. Excess amounts of omega 6 fatty acids create an omega 3 deficiency in of itself.

How to Incorporate More Omega 3 Fatty Acids
- Assess your fat/oil intake on a daily basis.
- Examine where your fat intake comes from, whether it comes from fats/oils, meat, fried foods, donuts, junk food, etc.
- Increase your omega 3 fatty acids by adding them to your daily diet. For example, make a salad with just flax seed oil or a combination of olive and flax oil together to increase your omega 3 intake while lowering your omega 6 fatty acids.
- Take supplements to offset other fats in your diet and bring

about the proper balance. For instance, supplement daily
with fish oils, flax seed oil or other comparable oils like hemp,
walnut or chia. (Look online for a full list of additional
options.) I personally feel supplements will be necessary to
achieve an optimum and healthy balance.

- Assess any intake of foods that retains oil, like potato chips,
corn chips, popcorn, processed foods, imitation cheese on
pizza, donuts or deep fried foods.
- Caution: Do not heat these oils (you may use them in or on
your food that has already been prepared).

What to Watch for When Buying Omega 3 Fatty Acid Supplements
- Do not buy omega 3, 6, and 9 combinations; buy only omega 3s.
- Potency is measured in milligrams; the balance of EPA to DHA
is predominately 2:1.
- Some brands advertise extra-high potency, but know that these
are just gimmicks. The ratio is always 2:1 of EPA to DHA; the
only deciding factor is the milligrams on the bottle. Companies
will charge up to four times more for their mock "extra-
strength" product.

Can I Get Enough Omega 3 Fatty Acids by Eating Fish?
The amount of fatty fish an average consumer eats would not produce the
health requirements suggested by health care professionals and researchers.

What About the Toxins in Fish and Supplements?
- Anyone who eats fish regularly has elevated levels of mercury.
The bigger the fish, the more mercury, PCBs and dioxins you
consume. Fish oil supplements are a cleaner source of omega 3
fatty acids. Most manufacturers today remove the mercury and
other toxic heavy metals from their products.
- Choose purity, potency and freshness: the brand you buy
should be able to provide you with a detailed biochemical and
toxicology analysis of its contents, be it in liquid or capsule form.

Vitamin D Benefits Crohn's Disease and Other Similar Complications

As human beings, it is our natural instinct to seek better health and longer
life. Every day, research is showing more and more benefits resulting from

the consumption of vitamins, minerals and other phytochemicals. The overall treatment mentality is slowly shifting to one of proactive habits, preventing illness before it occurs (as opposed to a treatment mentality focused on curing illnesses after they happen).

When looking at nutrients for building and maintaining the body, vitamin D holds a prominent place on the list of importance. Yet several aspects of culture and lifestyle are inhibiting the availability of this sunlight vitamin. Today, more and more adults are taking drastic measures to avoid the sun's UV rays. Once thought to be an uncommon condition of modern times, research has now shown that vitamin D deficiency is on the rise. People who fall into this category are those who work long hours in offices, or whose clothing and lifestyle keep them out of the sunlight. Also included are adults over 50, post-menopausal women, dairy intolerant individuals, anyone living in cold or northern regions, and those who overuse sunscreen.

The following section will delve into the complexities of vitamin D and its many applications, as it applies to our daily health. We will explore the hazards of vitamin D deficiencies, companion supplements, dietary sources, and appropriate dosages, including the various forms and their effectiveness.

Vitamin D Benefits Crohn's Disease

Exciting news arrived recently from a Canadian research study, headed by Dr. John White, an endocrinologist at the Research Institute of the McGill University Health Centre. Dr. White led a team of scientists from McGill University and the Université de Montréal in a study involving vitamin D and inflammatory bowel disease (IBD).

Their findings were extremely favorable, demonstrating the value of vitamin D as an inhibitor to Crohn's disease and as an anti-microbial agent. Dr. White states, "Our data suggests for the first time that vitamin D deficiency can contribute to Crohn's disease, especially in individuals who live in the northern hemisphere." Dr. White's findings kept bringing him back to the effect vitamin D had upon the immune system; in particular, the microbes within the gut. Dr. White says, "It's a defect in innate immune handling of intestinal bacteria that leads to an inflammatory response that may lead to an autoimmune condition." His suggested dosage is 1000 mg of vitamin D, twice a day.

Winter Blues

When winter is upon us, during the many days of reduced sunlight the lack of vitamin D poses a hazard to our health. In actual fact, getting adequate exposure to the sun's rays combats the condition SAD (seasonal affective disorder), sometimes called "winter blues." Published research shows that vitamin D is an important nutrient for our brain, as well as our body. In one such study, a mere five days of treatment with vitamin D (at a dosage of 400–800 IU per day) improved winter depression. Further research involving lengthier trials supported the link between vitamin D and moods, indicating the biochemical basis for SAD. So, whenever possible, make an effort to get outside— especially on bright days during the cold season.

Further Application of Vitamin D

A major application of vitamin D involves calcium absorption. It is virtually impossible for the body to properly assimilate calcium and phosphorus without vitamin D. When vitamin D supplies are insufficient, the body robs our bones for the calcium it needs. As a result, healthy bones and teeth will begin to fade away if levels of vitamin D are not sustained.

Ongoing research linking vitamin D deficiency and abnormal cell development, as seen in cancer cases, has shown great promise, particularly in the areas of colon, prostate and breast cancer. Vitamin D regulates the genes associated with cancers and autoimmune disease. Vitamin D also helps in the growth of new skin cells; distressing disorders such as psoriasis and other itchy, flaking problems have been helped with higher levels of vitamin D. In addition to inadequate sunlight, hereditary, kidney and liver disorders inhibit the absorption of vitamin D. Deficiency of vitamin D leads to impaired bone mineralization, contributing to bone softening diseases such as rickets, osteoporosis and osteomalacia.

Complexities of Vitamin D

Vitamin D3, also known as cholecalciferol, is a secosteroid structurally similar to steroids such as testosterone, cholesterol and cortisone. Cholecalciferol is the *only* natural form of vitamin D, manufactured in large quantities when our bare skin is exposed to the sunlight. All other forms are molecules that have vitamin D *activity*. Experts recommend a natural form of vitamin D, rather than synthetic. Vitamin D (25-dihydroxyvitamin D) in its active form is a hormone that binds to the body's cellular receptors.

Vitamin D2, or calciferol, promotes a healthy heart and thyroid, aids metabolism and promotes assimilation of calcium for healthy bone formation. Calciferol is *not* a naturally-occurring vitamin within humans. It is produced by radiating fungus, which form fat-like substances called ergocalciferol. Since this form of vitamin D is derived from plants, it is considered kosher.

Vitamin D is a Pre-Hormone, Not a Hormone
Similar to cholesterol, the body turns vitamin D into two hormones, calcidiol and calcitriol, which are collectively called vitamin D. For instance, the body uses cholesterol to make hormones such as estrogen and testosterone; in much the same way, cholecalciferol taken from our skin or supplements is turned into hormones by the body.

Importance of Calcitriol and Calcidiol
Calcitriol is the most potent steroid hormone in our bodies, a derivative of cholecalciferol, and is manufactured from calcidiol in our kidneys and tissues. Calcitriol blood levels refer to a vitamin D deficiency testing, the only one required.

How to Take Vitamin D
Vitamin D is a fat-soluble vitamin, requiring the presence of fat for best absorption (preferably mono and polyunsaturated fats) and should therefore always be taken with a meal.

Companion Supplements

- Calcium: promotes healthy teeth, gums, bones, neuromuscular activity, blood clotting
- Phosphorous: promotes healthy metabolic function, healthy bones and teeth
- Vitamin C: promotes healthy immune system, aids in formation of collagen and iron absorption, destroys free radicals
- Vitamin A: promotes healthy skin, hair, bones, eyes, immune system, embryonic development, nervous system, brain
- Iron and zinc: can be poorly regulated in the presence of vitamin D deficiency

---

Daily Dosage of Vitamin D (Recommended Dietary Allowance (RDA))
- For infants 0–6 months to 12 months: 400 IU
- For children 1–8 years: 600 IU
- For children, men and women aged 9–69: 600 IU
- Adults past the age of 70: 800 IU.

Note: In the absence of sunlight, 1000 IU of cholecalciferol is required for children and 4000 IU for adults.

Dietary Sources
Fatty fish are natural sources of vitamin D, such as catfish, mackerel, salmon, tuna in oil and sardines. Milk and grains are often fortified with vitamin D to minimize the risk of vitamin D deficiency.

Toxicity
The naturally rejuvenating benefits of vitamin D help our bodies remain strong, vibrant and resistant to damage. But overexposure to sunlight may result in vitamin D toxicity, affecting an individual's equilibrium leaving them light headed, what is sometimes referred to as sunstroke. The level of vitamin D found in normal food and supplements is too low to be toxic. An overdose of vitamin D usually occurs only when excessive doses of the prescription form are taken.

Supplementation Overview

Many with gastrointestinal disorders have difficulties involving malabsorption, and consequently become malnourished. Weight loss is standard in 65–75 percent of inflammatory bowel disorder patients (IBD). There are a variety of causes for this: difficulty eating around pain; diarrhea; anorexia and nausea; as well as inadequate diets without the support of supplementation.

Another common contributor is fat malabsorption, which results in substantial calorie depletion and loss of fat soluble vitamins and minerals. There can also be bile acid malabsorption, involving the ileum or resection of this area.

Other factors include the following:
- Bacterial overgrowth
- Drugs that depress protein synthesis, increasing nutritional needs of vitamins and minerals, decreasing bone formation, etc.

- Diarrhea, resulting in loss of nutrients and electrolytes
- Plasma and protein depletion
- Infection, inflammation and fever

For these reasons and more, I cannot overstress the importance of correcting nutritional deficiencies. A daily diet should consist of fruits, vegetables, nuts, cheeses and some animal products or vegetarian protein. It is possible to be a vegetarian, even though certain nutrients are harder to come by when on a strict vegetarian diet (for example, it is difficult to obtain sufficient iron and B12 when omitting animal products). Normally, soy products and soy milk are restricted on this diet; although, depending on individual intolerances and sensitivities, soy tofu and soy cheese are sometimes allowed. Supplements may be necessary to sustain adequate levels of iron and B12. Deficiency of vitamin B12 is widespread in Crohn's disease patients because absorption of this vitamin is suppressed by the disease's process in the lower part of the small intestine (ileum). All supplements must be checked for additives such as whey, lactose, starch, yeast and any unwanted chemicals.

Dr. Donovan suggests shiitake mushrooms, both for its beneficial antiviral effects and its ability to activate the immune system. He also recommends vitamin C at just below tolerance—in other words, the highest dose which does not cause diarrhea. Beta-carotene, zinc, and multi-vitamin and mineral supplements for the treatment of viral gastroenteritis is also suggested. Dr. Donovan states, "The advantage of vitamin A, zinc and beta-carotene, is that they help the lining of the gastrointestinal tract repair and regenerate itself very well."[8]

An essential staple in our diets, as we have learned through recent research, is fish oil. Fish oil houses the recommended combination of the fat soluble vitamins A and D. For some time, this supplement has proven helpful during winter months for those who live in northern regions. Wild salmon oil, cod liver oil, krill and other quality fish oil supplements should be at least at a recommended daily allowance of 400 IU vitamin D and 5000 IU vitamin A. If for some reason you cannot digest or tolerate the oil form of these nutrients, there are alternatives in the form of water soluble vitamins A and D; otherwise, enteric coated fish oil supplements (which stay intact until it reaches the intestine) may be an option.

---

8   Alternative Medicine (1994), Gastrointestinal Disorders, Deepak Chopra M.D., 680-689.

Certain nutrients can be taken in one tablet, such as B-complex vitamins, B12, B2, niacinamide, and B6. E. Gottschall advises, "Too much
folic acid should be avoided; the amount taken should range from about
0.1–0.8 mg. Folic acid and B12 work in unison in the cells of the body
and it is important not to take more than 0.4 mg folic acid unless one is
positive that B12 levels are in the high normal range; only then may one
take up to 0.8 mg."

Nutrient Loss Due to Medication and Diarrhea

Vitamin supplementation, specifically B-complex supplementation, needs
to be addressed among women who are on contraceptive medication, due
to the depleting effects caused by traditional birth control medication.
Vitamin C is a lost food element, enhanced by various methods of cooking
(or exposure to air), and is used up at a tremendous rate by the body if
one smokes tobacco. As long as diarrhea is not enhanced, a larger dose of
vitamin C with bioflavonoids is advisable; although, if diarrhea is present,
try 100 mg.

Through my practice and knowledge, I find it is extremely difficult for
people with intestinal problems to obtain adequate minerals, vitamins and
antioxidants through their diet alone, without incorporating supplements.
Electrolyte and trace mineral deficiencies are also typical in people with a
history of chronic diarrhea. In fact, patients suffering with inflammatory
bowel disease should be on a program of therapeutic vitamin supplements
at least five times the recommended daily allowance. Higher doses of minerals may also need to be added. Calcium and magnesium deficiencies may
be a result of chronic steatorrhea—abnormally increased amounts of fat
in the feces, brought on by the reduced absorption of fat in the intestine.

A List of Common Deficiencies

A lack of magnesium is a complication which may require intravenous
or injections to maintain even minimal levels. Magnesium taken intrave-
nously (at a dose of 200–400 mg) may be necessary when the patient does
not respond to oral supplementation. Oral supplementation of magnesium may need to be chelated otherwise, citrate or aspartate, rather than
inorganic magnesium salts such as carbonate.

Suggested Dosage: 300 mg, 1–3 times a day (taken with a protein source).

Zinc is another common deficiency, which is *crucial* for the immune system. In addition, low iron levels and anemia occur frequently as a result of inadequate amounts of B12 or folate (also through blood loss). Furthermore, other nutrients that usually run low and need attention are calcium, potassium, copper, niacin, vitamin A, vitamin D, vitamin E and vitamin K.

Digestive and Anti-Inflammatory Enzymes

Digestive enzymes have beneficial effects for IBD patients, celiac patients and on all forms of colitis and IBS, specifically in terms of aiding digestion while also alleviating pain and inflammation. Bromelain is a type of proteolytic enzyme (an enzyme that eats protein), which is normally taken to assist digestion. However, research has shown that bromelain can inhibit the cyclooxygenase enzyme, thereby relieving pain and inflammation. Proteolytic enzymes work best on an empty stomach for inflammation; otherwise, add a small amount of carbohydrate to buffer (but not protein). Papin and pancreatic enzymes are also anti-inflammatory and used to aid the digestive process. When using as a digestion enhancer, take digestive enzymes only as directed by the product's manufacturer.

Supplements with Wonderful Healing and Nourishing Properties

Chlorella: 18 mg to 3 gm daily in water or juice (taken as tablets or powder). This edible algae stimulates blood cleansing and feeds the friendly flora in the bowel. Chlorella is a whole food, containing rich sources of vitamins, minerals, enzymes, and is the highest known source of chlorophyll. Chlorella is very high in nucleic acids, provided by its concentration of RNA and DNA.

Acidophilus and **Bifidum (Probiotic):** Take as directed by the brand of choice. Probiotics repel detrimental bacteria in the gastrointestinal tract. Many factors adversely affect the immune system's defenses, some of which are the overuse of antibiotics, prescription drugs, stress and environmental pollutants like pesticides. If you have dairy intolerance, purchase a nondairy product.

Colostrum: Take two capsules twice a day (of quality product) for the repair of the intestinal lining and boosting the immune system. (Refer to Chapter 9 for the benefits of colostrum.)

Fish Oils: Fish oils supply lubrication and vitamins A and D, which are needed for healthy elimination. Research demonstrates the benefits of fish oil for Crohn's patients; over a twelve month study, it was shown that the agents in fish oil can minimize the inflammatory processes, which may prove beneficial in prolonging remission in patients with Crohn's disease.[9]

Ginseng: A traditional Chinese herb dating back more than 2,000 years, ginseng is known as an adaptogenic herb that has shown to increase vigor, stamina, resistance to infections and protection against environmental toxins and radiation. It is also very supportive to the male and female reproductive systems. For fatigue, take 500 mg, three times a day.

Ashwagandha: Ashwagandha is an adaptogenic herb with a lineage of over 3,000 years of use in traditional medicine. Of particular interest, ashwagandha inhibits the breakdown of acetylcholine, thereby combating stress. Clinical trials support its use in many health implications, such as neurological disorders, inflammation, nervousness, insomnia, cardiovascular protection, lowering blood glucose and cholesterol levels, normalizing hormones and battling oxidative stress. For neurological stress, take 500 mg, three times a day. For liquid extracts, take 25 ml three times a day.

Apple Cider Vinegar: A great cleanser of mucus and catarrhal conditions, apple cider vinegar is very high in potassium and helps provide nutrients needed by muscle tissues. Take 1–3 teaspoons in water two times a day.

Dulse: Very high in trace minerals not obtained from the soil, dulse stimulates the thyroid gland and speeds up the metabolism. The thyroid gland plays a part in bowel activity. Suggested Dosage: 500 mg, 1–3 times a day.

Evening Primrose Oil: This oil contains essential fatty acids (unsaturated), known for relieving inflammation, eczema and menopausal symptoms. Take two capsules 2–3 times a day with food.

Garlic Capsules (Kyolic): Take two yeast-free Kyolic capsules with meals. Garlic has a healing effect on the colon and is a natural antibiotic. Alternatively, add cloves of raw garlic to your daily diet in yogurt or use it in cooking. To retain its antibacterial properties, do not overcook garlic.

9 Belluzzi A, N Engl J Med 334, 1557-1560 (1996).

Rutin and **Quercetin:** These bioflavonoids offer several protective and healing benefits. They have been shown to significantly reduce bowel adhesions and intestinal surface damage. Rutin and Quercetin have a protective anti-inflammatory effect on the colon mucosal wall. Suggested dosage, coupled with vitamin C, is 500 mg, 2–3 times a day.

Aloe Vera Juice: Aloe vera enhances tissue repair of the intestinal tract and, when applicable, softens fecal matter. Consume ¼–½ cup, three times daily until improvement is noticed, and then reduce.

Apple Juice: Freshly prepared apple juice is high in pectin, which is a moisture-holding substance.

Herbs: Herbal supplements are very nourishing and healing complements for all gastrointestinal aliments. (Refer to Chapter 11: Herbal Recommendations.)

Tissue Salts

Tissue salts (also referred to as cell salts or biochemic salts) are simple minerals that our bodies require to maintain good health.

One of Hahnemann's (a pioneer of homeopathic medicine) early supporters, Dr. Wilhem Schüessler was a 19th century German doctor who discovered that when human body cells were reduced to ash, they contained 12 mineral salts. He became an early adapter of this new system of medicine and was instrumental in formulating tissue salts as nutritional therapy. He observed symptoms that occurred when there was a deficiency of certain tissue salts. Dr. Scheussler reasoned that the fastest way to resolve these symptoms was to ingest the salts orally by mouth for direct absorption into the body. He determined the proper dosage to be a 600 percent dilution. Similar to a homeopathic protocol, tissue salts are used as nutritional supplementation according to symptoms.

Tissue Mineral Salts

1. Calcium Fluoride
2. Calcium Phosphate
3. Calcium Sulphate

4. Iron Phosphate

5. Potassium Chloride

6. Potassium Phosphate

7. Potassium Sulphate

8. Magnesium Phosphate

9. Sodium Chloride

10. Sodium Phosphate

11. Sodium Sulphate

12. Silica

Tissue salts have become very popular and respected in their ability to work remarkably quickly and effectively. Tissue salts are generally available in two forms:

1. Minute amounts of the salt in a lactose-base soluble tablet.

2. Minute amounts of the salt in an alcohol-base, for those who are highly lactose-intolerant.

How to Take Tissue Salts

Place one or two tablets under the tongue and allow to fully dissolve. Tissue salts are absorbed into the bloodstream via the blood vessels under the tongue. If an alternative method is needed, the tablets can be crushed and dissolved in a little water. Mineral salts may be added to enema solutions or through feeding tubes, depending on the individual needs of the person. The liquid form of the salts, as a rule, is dissolved in water and consumed. Dissolve four tablets under tongue four times a day or hourly for acute episodes.

Notes on Tissue Salts

- Sodium sulphate is recommended for diarrhea when stools are green in color. This type of diarrhea is chronic, usually worse in the mornings or alternates with constipation.

- Potassium chloride for stools lighter in color; the tongue may have a whitish coating. Symptoms are aggravated by eating rich, creamy foods or pastries.

- Potassium sulphate for when stools are slimy and yellow in color with a great deal of gas and intermittent abdominal cramping.

- Potassium phosphate is helpful when diarrhea is accompanied with stress, fright and worry. Stools are very pungent with a golden yellow color—may contain blood.

- Magnesium phosphate is useful when the main problem is sharp cramping and gas. It can be used in combination with other tissue salts.

- Warm packs on the stomach area are helpful to aid digestion after meals.

What Vitamins and Minerals are Lost with Crohn's Disease, Colitis, Celiac, IBS and Chronic Diarrhea?

Inflammatory bowel disorders are extremely serious and involve nutrient deficiencies, marked by gut permeability and excessive loss of nourishment. Irritable bowel syndrome (IBS) may not fall under the same umbrella as the chronic conditions of Crohn's, colitis or celiac; however, nutrient loss and their suggested remedies have applications for all gut disorders. A prominent problem associated with Crohn's and ulcerative colitis is the malabsorption of the vital nutrients needed to sustain health while regenerating and repairing tissue throughout the intestinal lining. Physical factors, such as chronic diarrhea, lack of appetite, medications, surgically altered segments in the intestines and blunted intestinal villi, contribute to the malabsorption of nutrients.

The following is a list of nutrients most often found in insufficient amounts (with their primary functions):

Zinc: For sustaining and enhancing the healing process; all conditions of gut dysbiosis require appropriate amounts of zinc. In particular, Crohn's and ulcerative colitis patients have need of adequate and regular amounts of the mineral zinc. Zinc is the second most important element in our bodies, performing a hundred or more functions, among them tissue repair and immune function. Zinc is also a cofactor for more than 300 enzymes. This crucial trace mineral is a necessary component of our immune response and healing process.

Suggested Dosage: 30 mg, once a day (for males) and 25 mg once a day (for females). For acute symptoms, take twice a day until symptoms subside.

Glutamine: The amino acid L-glutamine plays an essential role, serving as the first line of defense in our intestines and the body as a whole. When deficient, this amino acid is implicated in immune dysfunction. Glutamine has particular benefits for gut complaints, for it is directly involved in the cell replication of the most rapidly multiplying cells in the body. Found in the intestines, these cells (called "enterocytes") are located in the mucosa lining of the small intestine. Through several metabolic steps leading up to the damage of the intestinal lining (mucosa), the demand for glutamine greatly increases. When supplies falter, the mucosal lining begins to break down. This is the process that sets up leaky or permeable gut.

Diarrhea causes a loss of electrolytes and water (among other nutrients) from the body. Glutamine has been shown to lessen the loss of these nutrients, along with enhancing the body's water and salt intake. The maintenance and support provided by glutamine carries on through to the large bowel, and has also been shown to assist in the healing of peptic stomach ulcers.

The applications of glutamine extend throughout the body where, among other processes, glutamine serves as an energy source for other rapidly dividing cells, such as immune cells following a bacterial invasion or other immune threat. Deficiencies occur following a trauma, major illness, poor diet and even excessive exercise. Glutamine is found abundantly in high protein foods such as meat, as well as being plentiful in two vegetable sources—uncooked cabbage and beets. Extra supplementation is recommended for problematic gut complaints.

Suggested Dosage: 250–500 mg, 1–3 times a day.

Magnesium: Vital for Crohn's, pancolitis, IBS, and many primary functions, magnesium is arguably the most important mineral in the body. Not only does magnesium assist in the production of cellular energy, but the heart cannot make use of the constant energy supply needed to function properly without adequate magnesium. A few other requirements of magnesium include energy production, bones and teeth, neuromuscular sensory systems and the synthesis of vitamin D (to assist calcium in finding its way into the bloodstream).

Magnesium is involved in many biological roles and performs more functions than any other mineral by a significant margin. It is the relaxer in the body, is routinely called upon by the downside of the heart beat, prevents muscles from cramping and works hand in hand with calcium for healthy bones and teeth. Magnesium can also be useful as a natural antispasmodic.

How to Take Magnesium

All minerals, including magnesium, require a protein to be ingested at the time of consumption. For example, small amounts of yogurt, ground flax seeds, nut butters, whey or other protein powders and meals where a portion includes protein. All other supplements are to be taken with food unless specified on the label.

Magnesium, like other minerals, requires an amino acid to carry and direct them onto their designated path throughout the body. For optimum absorption of this important mineral, supplementation is recommended to help safeguard against a shortage.

Since magnesium is the main element in the body, performing many more functions than any other, it is crucial that we ensure the availability of this mineral by way of supplementation.

Suggested Dosage: 300–500 mg, 1–3 times a day.

Why is Magnesium Important for Crohn's Disease and Similar Complications?

The carrier protein for magnesium is commonly impaired by conditions of Crohn's disease, often times with colitis, and occasionally with other gut abnormalities. Magnesium is used liberally throughout the body; when it becomes unavailable, metabolic functions requiring the mineral can cease. There is no doubt as to its fundamental role in the maintenance of the body and its further healing and balancing requirements. It is not uncommon for an unavailability of magnesium (brought on by malabsorption) to be the culprit in blocking a total disease reversal—something which has been particularly noted in chronic intestinal disorders. Regardless of your current health status, pay special attention to magnesium when you feel you are doing everything else right.

Vitamin C: Vitamin C reaches every cell of the body and plays a significant role in fighting infection by stimulating immune response (production of white blood cells) against the onslaught of disease causing invaders. Vitamin C is widely available in many fruits and vegetables.

Suggested Dosage: 500 mg, 1–3 times a day. Depending on symptoms, more may be required and doubling of the dosage is not uncommon. Purchase a non-acidic or more absorbable, gentler variety for the gut.

Vitamin D: Vitamin D is necessary, especially for those individuals taking corticosteroids. This vitamin is high on the list for people with Crohn's, ulcerative colitis and celiac diseases to maintain strong bones and prevent osteoporosis; in particular, those taking steroid type drugs. (Refer to "Vitamin D Benefits Crohn's Disease and Other Similar Complications" early in this chapter)

Calcium: Calcium is another bone mineral, which, like so many other minerals, is lost if diarrhea or internal bleeding are present. Calcium is also needed for cell membrane permeability and blood-clotting. Corticosteroids can reduce calcium levels; depending on absorption levels, calcium is best taken before bedtime or twice a day with food.

Suggested Dosage: 1000 mg, 1–2 times a day (for troublesome gut symptoms)

Folate: Folic acid and B12 are vitamins that perform similar function in our bodies: they are both required for holding iron in the blood. Folic acid is necessary for making red blood cells, and B12 is found in low amounts in Crohn's and other inflammatory bowel disorder patients. Supplemental or B12 injections are often required for anemia, digestive difficulties, fatigue and fetal development. Folic acid is necessary for DNA synthesis and the reproduction of all cells. Likewise, B12 is needed for DNA and RNA synthesis and is vital for production of every cell, particularly every red blood cell.

These vitamins work as a team for energy production, immune function and for sustaining a healthy nervous system. Furthermore, B12, folic acid and vitamin C, allow the body to use proteins.

Suggested Dosage: A blood test will more clearly determine dosage requirements. Otherwise, 1200 mcg of B12 under the tongue is advisable. Support formulas may contain both nutrients.

Vitamin K: Crohn's and other similar disorders have a history of bleeding and gut permeability. Vitamin K is best known for its role in maintaining healthy blood clotting. Our body has the ability to manufacture vitamin K in the form of K2, produced by our intestinal bacteria, while K1 is found in plants. Vitamin K is plentiful in chlorophyll. Because of the nature of gut dysbiosis disorders, vitamin K may be required in supplementation.

Suggested Dosage: 500–1000 mcg of K2 once a day.

Omega 3 Fatty Acids: These essential nutrients do not actually fall under the label of vitamin or mineral, but do contribute a great deal to the healing process. EFAs reduce inflammation, especially when in the form of fish oil. Omega 3 fatty acids, derived from flax seeds, are short chain fatty acids. The brain only utilizes long chain fatty acids like those found in fish oil; therefore, I always recommend regular supplementation of fish oil to help with the many complications resulting from memory problems and other cognitive disabilities. For vegetarians and vegans, refer to the beginning of this chapter for recommendations to ensure adequate intake of omega 3 fatty acids for optimum health.

Suggested Dosage: 1000 mg, 1–3 times a day.

Homocysteine: Homocysteine is a naturally occurring toxic amino acid which is converted into the amino acid methionine under normal conditions. This metabolic pathway is a process known as methylation. An unhealthy diet and lifestyle interferes with methylation and leads to an unhealthy build-up of homocysteine.

CHAPTER ELEVEN

Natural Remedies and Formulas for Healing Intestinal Tract Tissue

Herbal Recommendations

Medicinal plants are a major component of medicine which has become even more relevant today than it ever was in ancient times. As a healing therapy, herbs dominate the list of remedies used throughout China (as in trimethylglycine), India (as in Ayurvedic medicine), and in European and Native American traditions. Many natural extracts from plants have found their way into mainstream medicines. These substances and their derivatives are the source for thousands of drugs and medicines worldwide.

However, an isolated and compounded element being *sourced* from plants (such as is found in manufactured medicine) does not imply that they are all safe. When isolated from the balancing principles within the plant itself and concentrated, the isolated component produces an overwhelming effect upon the body.

A few examples of plant extracts made into popular medications include morphine, reserpine, digitoxin, vincristine and vinblastine, all of which are toxic in a concentrated form.

Other examples of plants and herbs being used for medicinal purposes include:

- Serpina: Used as a sedative, seprina is the original tranquilizing drug, derived from Rauwolfia serpentina (due to the alkaloid reserpine)
- Vincristine: A chemotherapy agent developed from rosy periwinkle
- Paclitaxel (Taxol): A chemotherapy agent derived from the Pacific yew Taxus brevifolia
- Vinblastine and vincristine: Used to treat leukemia and Hodgkin's disease, and extracted from the Madagascar periwinkle
- Papaver somniferum: A pain killer/morphine equivalent to the opium poppy
- Heart medicine Digitalis: Purple Foxglove, is the source of digitoxin, a cardiac drug
- White willow bark: A popular and non-toxic replacement for aspirin

When referencing herbs or phytochemistry and the science of herbology, these terms refer to the parts of plants used as a healing therapy for their nourishing and balancing properties. The numerous plant-based therapies throughout this book will demonstrate the effectiveness of whole plants for treating the many chronic and acute conditions that routinely plague mankind. These recommendations involve the above-ground, aerial plant parts such as leaves, bark, stems and flowers, and the below-ground root portion of the plant. The delicate parts of plants, including the leafy parts and flower, follow the process for steeped tea called an infusion. The hard woody and fibrous parts, such as the bark and roots, require a decoction process.

How to Make an Infusion or Decoction

Infusion: An infusion is another word for tea. To make tea, add 1–2 teaspoons of herb to 1 cup of boiling water. Steep for 15 minutes. Strain and serve warm for medicinal purposes, the preferred method to impart healing of intestinal tissue.

Decoction: The hard or woody parts of the plant require a different process in order to pull out sufficient healing properties. The root, bark and other hard plant substances require a light boiling method. The herb of choice should already be broken down into a powder for best results. Mix 1 teaspoon of dried herb or 3 teaspoons of fresh herb to one cup of water into a pot. Bring a pot of water to a boil (never use aluminum pots) and simmer for 10–15 minutes. Strain and serve as suggested for infusion method.

Combination Tea for an Infusion/Decoction Blend: Follow decoction directions for the root or woody parts of the formula. When the decoction process is finished, add the aerial parts to the existing tea blend and steep for a further 15 minutes.

Healing Properties of Herbs

Demulcent herbs soothe and relieve irritated, inflamed mucous membranes. They have a slippery, protective quality while applying lubrication to tissue surfaces.

Examples include:

- Marshmallow
- Comfrey
- Slippery Elm
- Licorice
- Mullein
- Flax seed
- Coltsfoot
- Lungwort Moss
- Hops
- Iceland Moss

Astringent herbs have the ability to contract cellular walls, restricting unwanted discharge such as body fluids or blood.

Examples include:

- Argimony
- Meadowsweet
- Oak Bark
- Bayberry
- Cranesbill
- Pilewort
- Tormentil
- Lady's Mantle

The Benefits of Herbal Remedies

Celiac Disease
The goal of using herbal remedies for celiac disease is to help soothe intestinal inflammation and irritation, along with healing damaged mucous

membranes. Typically, celiac patients are overrun with candidia in the intestinal tract. The remedies for yeast and fungal growth can be seen in Chapter 7 (for destroying pathogens) and Chapter 9 (for protocols to control candidia and the benefits of probiotics).

In treating celiac disease, the focus is on repairing the intestinal tract, stimulating beneficial gut flora and killing candidia, while the diet remains gluten-free. The protein gluten triggers the body to produce antibodies that attack the *villi* in the small intestine, damaging its surface and resulting in pain, bloating, diarrhea and various other symptoms.

There are many suggestions in this book for herbal remedies to treat all the symptoms a celiac patient might encounter. For example, the following suggestions have proven helpful:

- Licorice root: soothing and demulcent; aids digestion
- Papin: aids digestion; take 500–1000 mg, with each meal
- Marshmallow root: soothes and controls inflammation
- Slippery elm: demulcent; nourishing; astringent; heals sores and reduces inflammation. Take 1 teaspoon herb powder taken in liquid, 3–5 times a day; or, make into a tea and sip throughout the day. When taking in capsule form, take 1000 mg, 3–5 times a day. May also be eaten by the spoonful mixed with hot liquid.
- Horsetail: very high in the mineral silicon (silica). Reduces inflammation and rebuilds/strengthens connective tissue. Dosage suggestion: Two 500 mg capsules, 3 times a day.
- Agrimony tincture: take 10 drops in water three times a day for any bouts of bleeding and diarrhea. Higher dosages may be required, such as 15–25 drops, taken several times a day until symptoms subside.
- Aloe vera: for intestinal repair; refer to Chapter 9 for further recommendations
- Apple pectin: soothing and healing
- Vitamin A, E, folic acid and zinc: are usually in demand for healing.
- Garlic, colloidal silver and grapefruit extract: for yeast and pathogens
- Dandelion: drink fresh as juice or powdered root in capsules; suggested dosage is 500 mg, taken 3 times a day.

Inflammatory Bowel Disease (IBD)

The classic herbal concoction known as Robert's Formula is an old sailor's remedy for inflammation and gut pain, which has since been updated and revised for use in healing inflammation associated with Crohn's disease, ulcerative colitis, and other gut complaints with similar symptoms. This modified formula is known as Bastyr's Formula, after John Bastyr, the naturopath responsible for the modifications. The updated recipe contains an animal extract of duodenal tissue, and is therefore not vegetarian. Several plant formulas such as Bastyr's and Roberts offer the benefit of flavonoids.

Patients with Crohn's disease, ulcerative colitis and chronic diarrhea suffer from nutrient deficiency. Subsequently, several plant flavonoids were included in Bastyr's Formula to enhance the immune system and support the healing process. The immune system is prompted into action when quercetin and other flavonoids react with enzymes influenced by processes associated with the inflammation response. Scavenger cells called macrophages and leucocytes remove bacteria and foreign material from the blood and provide protection against foreign invaders while assisting antibody production.

Bastyr's Formula

- 8 parts marshmallow root: relieves gastritis, ulcers, inflammation, and soothes high mucilage content

- 4 parts wild indigo: for intestinal infections, inflammation, anti-microbial, anti-catarrhal

- 8 parts echinacea (combined with goldenseal): antibacterial, supports the immune system and may be used to replace antibiotics

- 8 parts American cranesbill: improves diarrhea, stops bleeding, and is used in cancer treatment

- 8 parts goldenseal: relieves inflammation of the digestive system, antiviral in nature

- 8 parts poke root: heals ulcerations of the intestinal lining; also a strong remedy for edema

- 8 parts slippery elm: demulcent, relieves gastrointestinal inflammation, soothes inflamed mucous membrane lining of the digestive system

- 8 parts comfrey: rapid healing power of tissue and bone, due to allantoin, a cell proliferant, demulcent, anti-inflammatory, pain relieving and enhances the growth of connective tissue
- 8 parts cabbage powder: heals gastrointestinal ulcers
- 2 parts pancreatin: aids in the digestive process, a proteolytic enzyme
- 1 part niacinamide: anti-inflammatory, non-flushing vitamin B3
- 2 parts duodenal substance: heals gastrointestinal ulcers; animal extract, not vegetarian

How to Buy or Make a Combination Tea Formula Using Above- and Below-Ground Plant Material

Bastyr's Formula may be purchased in capsules by various herbal manufacturers. You may also buy these herbs loose and make your own capsules, or combine in a tea formula. If you choose to make your own tea, follow the directions for decoction when using root herbs, and infusion for aerial parts.

Dosage recommendation: 2–3 capsules with each meal until flare-up subsides; following a remission, reduce to 1 capsule, twice a day for a few months. This formula is often sold as Robert's Formula or Bastyr's Formula.

Additional Herbal Recommendations and Sample Formulas

Crohn's Disease and Ulcerative Colitis
- Comfrey root and leaf: Rapid healing of tissue throughout the body, such as bone and lining of the intestinal tract, due to its cell replication enhancing property (allantoin). A first choice for healing and diminishing the gut symptoms of Inflammatory Bowel Disorders (IBD) and other similar complaints. Drink 1 cup three times a day until healed. As a tincture extract, take 15 drops three times a day.
- Argimony extract or powder: Used to treat diarrhea and bleeding. Xian He Cao (Argimony grass) is astringent, coagulant, vermifuge, anti-cancer, cholagogue, emmenagogue, adult and child incontinence. Refer to Chapter 5 for how to treat diarrhea. Child dosages can be seen further into this chapter.

- Artichoke leaf extract: Symptoms of IBS and GERD (gastroesophageal reflux disease) were improved in clinical trials, and patients found it enhanced their quality of life through lower incidence of irritable bowels.
- Echinacea: Anti-bacterial and anti-fungal properties.
- Cat's claw: Fights inflammation.
- Garlic: A potent chemical called allicin is extracted from garlic, and which holds an amazing track record for destroying even the most antibiotic-resistant strains of bacteria.
- Goldenseal root: Anti-microbial and anti-viral action.
- Marshmallow root or leaf: Soothes the mucous membrane and promotes healing.
- Pau d'arco: Anti-bacterial, anti-fungal, bitter tonic, digestive aid.
- Rose hips: Nourishing, mild diuretic, mild laxative, astringent qualities.
- Slippery elm: Promotes healing of intestinal tract lining and reduces inflammation.
- Yerba mate: Carminative.
- Turkish Rhubarb: Anti-bacterial and anti-viral properties; good for constipation and diarrhea. An important part of Chinese formulas for treating fever.
  - Low dosage for diarrhea: ½ teaspoon dried herb root extract; make a decoction and strain. Drink 1 cup three times a day. Higher dosages become purgative, and good for constipation.
- Sheep sorrel: Anti-cancer and tumor properties; astringent, mild laxative, for sores and inflammation. A main ingredient in essiac tea.
  - Dosage suggestion: 500 mg, taken three times a day.
- Burdock root: For blood purifying and reducing inflammation.
  - Dosage suggestion: 200 mg, taken three times a day.
- Humic acid: This substance is not a single acid, but rather a complex formula of different acids found in nature. It is part of the organic constituent of soil. Humic acid is not well known as a nutritional supplement but is making itself known for its poly-electrolytes, which are unique colloids that diffuse easily through tissue membranes.

Herbal Formula that Successfully Replaced Prednisone
The plant sophora offers a wide range of benefits for healing, such as:
- Sophorae injection is shown to reduce the toxicity and harmful effects caused by chemotherapy drugs.
- Matrine, the main extract that is isolated from *Sophora flavescens*, has displayed anti-cancer activity in several types of cancer cells.
- Sophora is an anti-inflammatory and an antioxidant and effective against atopic dermatitis.
- It is suggested that this herb may have applications as a treatment for mast cell-derived allergic inflammatory diseases.

The following tea formula is very beneficial for diarrhea and fistulas in the anal region:
Tea Formula

Ling Zhi–Reishi Mushroom
Ku Shen–Sophora Root
Gan Cao–Licorice

The ratio consisted of:
20 grams of Ling Zhi – Reishi Mushroom
9 grams of Gan Cao – Sophora Root
3 grams of Ku Shen–Licorice

- 4.745 grams = 1 teaspoon
- 20 grams = 4¼ teaspoons
- 3 grams = 0.632 of a teaspoon
- 9 grams = 1.897 teaspoons

Dong quai is reported to be an excellent alternative to prednisone. Chinese herbs can be purchased online or from health stores that specialize in the sale of herbs. Herbal and supplement sources can be found at the end of this chapter.

Colitis
Colitis may be characterized by alternating bouts of constipation and diarrhea. A choice combination formula for this condition (or any similar complaint) would incorporate several different actions and qualities for

maximum benefit. For instance, herbs such as marshmallow and comfrey have demulcent qualities. Astringent action is found in bayberry, agrimony and also comfrey. For an anti-inflammatory, choose wild yam or bowsellia.

Herbs in the Form of Tea or Extract that Benefit Colitis

Boswellia	Cranesbill
Chamomile	Comfrey
Holy Basil	Dandelion
Garlic	Feverfew
Papaya	Periwinkle
Red clover	Shepherd's purse
Yarrow	Pau d'arco

Lobelia tea: Drink 1–3 cups per day. This may be used as an enema for inflammation of the colon.

Comfrey leaf, or root capsules and pepsin, partner well together during flare-ups. Take two capsules of comfrey and one of pepsin twice daily.

For gentle healing, mix one cup of fruit juice (made from fruits that are allowed) or vegetable juice, combined with ¼ cup aloe vera juice and take before meals.

Sample Formula for Crohn's Disease and Colitis

1 part comfrey root powder or leaf (root is preferable)
1 part slippery elm bark powder

This is a first-choice combination for Crohn's and colitis conditions, especially when accompanied by diarrhea or bleeding and particularly upon first initiating a healing program. Drink three cups throughout the day. The natural sweeteners stevia and raw honey may be added. Reduce once symptoms have significantly improved. Integrate the tea formula while correcting all nutritional deficiencies and any other remedy that may be required for additional associated symptoms, such as chronic diarrhea and anxiety.

Sample Formula for Colitis

3 parts wild yam	1 part echinacea
2 parts bayberry	1 part marshmallow root
1 part agrimony	½ part goldenseal
1 part comfrey	

Follow the instructions at the start of this chapter for making an infusion, decoction or a combination of both for herbal blend remedies

Anxiety or Agitation

If symptoms such as these are a concern, add herbs like valerian, skullcap and passionflower to the formula in one or two part additions. Refer to Chapter 8 for suggestions and remedies for depression, stress and anxiety.

Bulgarian Ulcerative Colitis Herbal Formula

A small yet relevant study took place in Bulgaria during 1982, involving 24 ulcerative colitis participants. The case subjects took an herbal combination formula consisting of dandelion, St. John's wort, lemon balm, calendula and fennel. By day 15, surprising results were seen in 23 out of 24 patients. The benefits included a complete remission of pain in the colon, a cessation of diarrhea and normalized fecal matter. The herb boswellia would be a welcome addition to further assist in reducing inflammation. Dosage of the above formula is 1 teaspoon (5 ml) three times daily in a little water before meals.

Boswellia Serrata

When results were compared side by side, the anti-inflammatory action of the herb boswellia was as effective as the drug sulphasalazine. Among other applications, boswellia has been shown to reduce inflammation when taken a few times a day as a tea or in some other preparation. It also works as an addition to a healing herbal formula.

Suggested Dosage: 500 mg, 3–6 times a day. When taken as a tea, take one cup 3–6 times a day. Reduce according to benefit.

Aloe Vera

Take ½ cup of aloe vera juice in the morning and at bedtime. Aloe vera's properties have proven beneficial in healing the colon and easing pain. Reduce dosage (if not well-tolerated) until improvement becomes evident.

Retention Enemas Provide Healing

Retention enemas have proven very useful for lower bowel inflammation, fistulas, abscesses, and other associated problems of gut disorders. Prepared solutions may be applied directly into the body by an enema bulb or another similar tool to evoke direct healing of inflamed colon tissue. The frequency of applications and the time duration (of retaining the enema solutions within the colon) will vary from person to person, depending on their individual tolerance and healing requirements.

Initially, these treatments should seek to soothe and calm the colon surface. There are several plant and herbal substances to choose from, which are used in accordance to the patient's receptivity to the solution. Herbs would be the safer choice as a first step over a whole plant (such as aloe vera) especially when the colon is very sensitive or inflamed.

For instance, comfrey root is a great healer with high mucilage content. Slippery elm and marshmallow root may be mixed with comfrey to impart further soothing and healing qualities, all of which fall under the decoction process, in terms of preparation. Use 1 teaspoon of powdered herb to 1 cup of water. Follow the decoction method found at the beginning of this chapter for making enema solutions. Typically, 1 pint (500 ml) is well-tolerated and comfortable. Hold the solution for 30 minutes; for lighter symptoms, start with 1–3 enemas per week and work upwards if they are proving to be beneficial in lowering associated symptoms of inflammation.

For IBD symptoms involving the anus, sigmoid colon and descending colon regions, daily application of retention enemas has shown to be highly beneficial for more immediate relief (when pain, inflammation, diarrhea and bleeding is related to these areas).

Retention Enema Formula for Colitis
When preparing a retention enema for colitis, begin by adding equal parts of comfrey root and slippery elm bark to a decoction tea process (one teaspoon of each herb mixed with 2–3 cups of boiling water). When bleeding is present, add five drops of agrimony tincture and cool to body temperature. This mixture becomes more gelatinous the longer it sits.

Insert enema solution into the rectum and lower colon region and hold for 30 minutes, and then eliminate. Repeat daily for chronic conditions and to promote a quicker initial healing (when the lower portion of the colon is involved with symptoms of bleeding, pain and inflammation). Note that these may be associated with colitis. Once bleeding has ceased, omit the argimony tincture. If a tincture product cannot be found, add argimony herb to the comfrey and slippery elm tea.

To promote further healing of the whole intestinal tract, ingest 1 cup of this tea formula (with or without an astringent herb like agrimony) three times a day along with the enema process. Additional herbal choices are marshmallow root, chamomile flowers, slippery elm powder (bark), or any herb that has a compatible action or property.

Aloe vera gel mixed with water is another great choice, although aloe vera is not always initially tolerated when there has been a prolonged incidence of gut inflammation. To be safe, wait 2–3 months before trying aloe vera as part of a retention enema solution.

For celiac patients who do not routinely deal with the symptoms of bleeding and diarrhea, the same formula of comfrey leaf or root and slippery elm bark (singularly or together) will assist in healing the mucosal intestinal tract lining.

Other substances can be added to the enema solution, such as tissue salts or liquids that destroy bacteria, like colloidal silver or tinctures that have anti-bacterial qualities (even garlic).

Another suggestion for relieving pain is adding white willow bark tea to the enema formula.

Butyrate Enema

Evidence suggests a link between impaired metabolism of the fatty acid butyrate and patients with ulcerative colitis.[10] Significant improvements and even remission were seen in 51 patients who were in an acute flare-up stage during a trial which involved butyrate retention enemas, applied twice daily for several weeks. Natural promoters of butyrate fatty acid include the fiber psyllium seed and butter (either clarified or ghee). Look for butyrate enema kits at pharmacies and health food stores.

Acupuncture

Patient testimonials, as well as research studies utilizing acupuncture, have demonstrated success in alleviating symptoms of Crohn's disease. Patients have found relief through Moxibuston, a process using the herb mugwort, which is burned over specific acupuncture points to penetrate more deeply into the body than needles alone.

Diarrhea (Adults)

The property to look for when seeking help from plants for problems

---

10 Roediger 1980; Chapman et al. 1994; Chapman et al. 1995; Thomas et al. 1996; Burke et al. 1997; Finnie et al. 1995; and Christl et al. 1996

involving diarrhea is the astringent quality, or the ability to contract cellular walls. Tannins are a component in herbs that cause an astringent action. It also causes a cotton-like feel in the mouth when drinking these teas. For example, black tea is loaded with tannins. Tea should be consumed every hour until symptoms subside. The following herbs are very helpful for diarrhea symptoms: agrimony, bayberry, bistort, black catechu, comfrey, cranesbill, meadowsweet, oak bark, plantain, rhatany, silverweed and tormentil.

Argimony is a first-choice herb that works well on its own, but which may also be coupled with other plants for their healing aspects, such as those that soothe and calm. The aerial parts of argimony are used in all forms of preparation, such as tinctures, capsules and loose herb. The tincture form will be the most potent in its concentration. For treating diarrhea and bleeding, take as often as needed.

In the beginning, depending on severity and frequency of symptoms, it would not be uncommon to take 10–15 drops four times over the first hour or two. Refer to the Initial Quick Start Program in Chapter 5 for more detailed information and suggestions on how to treat diarrhea and bleeding.

A sample formula of these first choice herbs is equal parts bayberry, cranesbill, meadowsweet and oak bark. Other good choices include avens, blessed thistle, burr-marigold, caraway, catnip, cinnamon, coriander, daisy, eyebright, ground ivy, jambul and kola.

Diarrhea (Children)
A gentle herbal preparation is called for in treating infants and young children. A go-to first herb is meadowsweet, because it is safe and may be used in all cases of diarrhea. Another good choice to accompany this herb is Lady's mantle. Mix equal parts using an infusion method and sweeten with honey, stevia or brown sugar if desired.

Diverticulitis
Psyllium seeds are an effective treatment for diverticuli, as they cleanse and soften the stool. Mullein, when used with other herbs, may also be helpful in the treatment of diverticulosis. Alfalfa, cayenne, chamomile, garlic, papaya, red clover and yarrow extract for tea is also good for diverticulitis.

The following is a sample formula for diverticulitis, a combination of demulcent, carminative, anti-spasmodic properties that serves as a welcome addition in soothing diverticulitis in its inflamed state. Make as a combination tea and drink 3–4 cups a day.

3 parts wild yam	1 part marshmallow
2 parts german chamomile	1 part ginger
1 part calamus	¼ part senna

Alfalfa

Alfalfa tablets contain all the fiber elements from the stems and leaves. Crack one or two tablets between the teeth and swallow with liquid at each meal. These tablets offer a type of fiber that isn't mucilage-forming in consistency. Alfalfa is especially recommended when implementing a cleansing type program or treating diverticulitis. The bulk fiber from alfalfa tablets works its way into the sacs or pouches (diverticuli), aiding in the removal of waste material. It is also high in vitamin K, a required element for healing.

Suggested Dosage: 500 mg (two tablets) twice a day.

Irritable Bowel Syndrome

While a complete treatment program for IBS can be found in Chapter 12, we'll lightly touch on a few plant extracts that can be beneficial as supplements. Peppermint is a natural antispasmodic, and peppermint tea has been shown to be quite effective in relieving abdominal pain. Peppermint oil is used in Europe, and enteric coated peppermint capsules are widely available. Take one at a time, as needed.

Other herbal recommendations include cascara sagrada (only for constipation), chamomile, lobelia, pau d' arco, and rose hips. When anxiety and stress accompany diarrhea, add herbs that calm and relax the person while relieving symptoms associated with IBS. Good choices include passionflower, skullcap, valerian and St. John's wort. (Refer to Chapter 8 for suggestions and remedies for depression, stress and anxiety).

Caution: Check the action of the herb before ingesting to ensure it relates to the desired symptom. For example, cascara sagrada is a strong laxative herb.

Determining Dosages for Children

There are several different techniques for determining the proper dosage for a child. Similar to parents who have grown accustomed to the needs and peculiarities of each of their children, most herbalists rely on years of experience and intuition when assigning dosages. When I recommend herbs for small children, I base my suggestions on the child's size, his or her general constitution, the nature of the illness, and the *herbs best suited for their action upon the body*. If you are newly introduced to herbal medicine and are not familiar with dosages, the following tables will be a great help in determining dosages. They provide sound guidelines for prescribing the proper amount of herbal preparation for children of all ages.

Nevertheless, remember that these tables are simply guidelines; it is equally important to factor in the weight and overall health of the child. Also consider the nature and severity of the illness and the quality and strength of the herbs being used. These are all important considerations, especially if you are using stronger herbs in a child's formula.

Suggested Dosages for Children

Here are some examples to assist in choosing an appropriate dosage:

WHEN ADULT DOSAGE IS 1 CUP (8 OUNCES OR 250 ML)	
AGE	DOSAGE
2–4 years	½–1 teaspoon
4–7 years	2–3 teaspoons
7–11 years	2 tablespoons

WHEN ADULT DOSAGE IS 1 TEASPOON, OR 60 GRAINS/DROPS	
AGE	DOSAGE
Younger than 3 months	2 grains/drops
3–6 months	3 grains/drops
6–9 months	4 grains/drops
9–12 months	5 grains/drops
12–18 months	7 grains/drops
18–24 months	8 grains/drops
2–3 years	10 grains/drops
3–4 years	12 grains/drops
4–6 years	15 grains/drops
6–9 years	24 grains/drops
9–12 years	30 grains/drops

Administering Herbal Medicine to Infants

Mother's milk is the safest and most effective way to administer herbs to infants. It is necessary for the mother to drink at least 4–6 cups of tea daily before the benefits will be imparted to the infant. Not only will the baby have the benefits of the gentle healing herbs, but the mother will as well. If a mother is not nursing, herbal teas and tinctures can be added directly to the baby's bottle.

Determining Dosages by Young's and Cowling's Rules

In determining the dosage for a child, consider the age, weight and the overall health of the child. These rules for determining dosage rely on mathematical calculations based on the child's age.

Young's Rule: Add 12 to the child's age. Divide the child's age by this total. For example, the dosage for a four-year old is 4÷16 = .25, or ¼ of the adult dosage.

Cowling's Rule: Divide the number of the child's next birthday by 24. For example, the dosage for a child who is three, about to turn four years old would be 4÷24 = .16, or approximately ¼ of the adult dosage.

| A TINCTURE EXAMPLE ||
| (WHEN AN ADULT DOSE IS 1 TEASPOON OR 60 DROPS): ||
AGE	DOSAGE
3–6 months	2 drops
6–9 months	4 drops
12–18 months	7 drops
2–3 years	10 drops
4–6 years	15 drops
9–12 years	30 drops

Illness rarely just occurs. Usually, it is a result of a stressed immune system, emotional imbalance, lack of sleep and poor nutrition. It may be a result of the child not keeping up with good hygiene, which lowers overall immunity protection. Sometimes illness occurs because the child is just having too much fun whirling through life. By closely observing the child, a parent or caregiver can usually detect the subtleties apparent when children become stressed, more anxious or seemingly out of balance, all of which may indicate susceptibility to illness. Children live passionately, and require an abundance of energy to maintain their typical activity level. This sustained state of energy output can leave even the most exuberant youngster exhausted and depleted.

All children are born with inherent strengths and weaknesses. Watch for these patterns early in life. Pay close attention to the energy levels of your child. Observe their health patterns throughout the year, and note which seasons brings special challenges for your child. Monitor and mentally log when or to what your child is most susceptible. This will help you become more aware of their health patterns.

The above information is provided in the hopes of expanding your knowledge and awareness of "choice" in treating children (and the family as a whole) as they make their way from infancy to adolescence. The objective is that this guidance will serve to ease the burden of common childhood illnesses, without building a foundation for future ones. The intention is *not* to replace the professional advice of a holistic health care practitioner or a family physician, but rather to complement such services.

Herbal and Supplement Product Sources and Locations

Manta (www.manta.com)
Manta has 21,806 companies under health food stores in the United States.

ACS (www.allcosmeticsource.com)
A source for all herbs in this book, including comfrey and agrimony flower extract (in powder form). A one world, one price provider which sells worldwide.

California Xtracts (www.californiaxtracts.com)
A source for comfrey liquid extract.

Frontier Co-op (www.frontiercoop.com)
Source for all herbs in this book.
Email: customercare@frontiercoop.com
Phone: 800-669-3275
Fax: 800-717-4372

Herb Pharm (www.herbpharm.com)

Source for comfrey extract, meadowsweet, marshmallow, adrenal and thyroid tincture support.

Christopher's Original Formula
Contains comfrey; available through numerous online retailers, including Amazon.com.

Solaray Products
Comfree, or Comfree Pepsin with Algin are products which, while they do not contain comfrey, still provide the naturally occurring aliantoin and mucilage—the desired compounds in comfrey.

Sangsters (www.sangsters.com)
Comfrey root powder and other herbal supplements.

Clef Des Champs Herbs (www.clefdeschamps.net)
Lady's mantle tincture and comfrey tincture.

Nelson Bach Flower Remedies (www.nelsonsnaturalworld.com, www.nelsonsstore.com)
Source for argimony extract.

Apotheke Herbal and Fruit Teas (www.docsimon.com)
Source for agrimony.

Eclectic Institute (www.eclectichrtb.com)
Extensive list of herbal and natural products

Nutraceutical Solaray (www.nutraceutical.com/collections/healthy/solaray)
Along with other companies under their umbrella, they are a good source for herbal supplements.

Solaray Alphabetical Product List (www.affordablesolaray.com/alpha-betical_listings.html)
Very long list of vitamins, minerals, supplements and herbals.

St. Frances Herb Farm (www.stfrancisherbfarm.com)
Located in Canada, along with three locations in the United States.

Botanica (TallGrass) (www.botanicahealth.com)

Vitamin Shoppe (www.vitaminshoppe.com)
Locations throughout the USA, with a few locations in Canada. Large selections of herbal products and quality nutraceuticals/supplements.

Boiron (www.boironusa.com)
Homeopathy resource.
Telephone: 1-800-264-7661

Now Foods (www.nowfoods.com)

Natural Factors (www.naturalfactors.com)

Orange Naturals (www.orangenaturals.com)
Professional products (Canada and international orders)

Goodness Me! Natural Food Market (www.goodnessme.ca)
Large selection of brand name products (herbal and supplements and organic food)

---

iHerb (www.iherb.com) Brands of Higher Concentration of Herbal Products and Supplement Products

California Xtracts	Herb Pharm	Nature's Way
Doctor's Best	Himalaya Herbals	Now Foods
Eclectic Institute	Jarrow Formulas	Paradise Herbs
Frontier Natural Products	Life Extension	Planetary Herbals
	Natural Factors	Source Naturals
Gaia Herbs	Nature's Answer	

Brands of Higher Concentration of Nutraceuticals/Supplements and Herbs

21st Century Health	Healthy Origins	Now Foods
California Gold Nutrition	Life Extension	Professional Brands
	Madre Labs	Quest Nutrition
Carlson Labs	Natrol	Rainbow Light
ChildLife	Natural Factors	Solgar
Country Life	Nature's Answer	Source Naturals
Doctor's Best	Nature's Plus	Thorne Research
Enzymedica	Nature's Way	ZOI Research
Garden of Life	Nordic Naturals	

See Chapter 14 for a list of resources for further information on herbal remedies.

CHAPTER TWELVE

Specific Dietary Protocols for Gastrointestinal Diseases

Acid and Alkaline Forming Foods for Typical Intestinal Disorders

Any dietary therapy should have as its complement a proper understanding of acidic and alkaline foods, to better facilitate the healing process. Aside from intestinal problems, having the correct proportions of acid to alkaline foods is essential for any individual striving to obtain and sustain a healthy way of life.

The proper pH blood balance is 80 percent alkaline and 20 percent acid. The body's pH levels are more acidic in the morning and become more alkaline throughout the day.

Protein and the Parathyroid Gland

Ideally, your pH levels should be in the range of 7.3 to 7.5. To briefly explain how the body achieves this optimum state, the parathyroid gland that sits on the thyroid gland controls the pH levels of the blood. Interestingly, this small, hard-working gland never stops doing its job, no matter what its actions affect. But this isn't always such a good thing; one such scenario occurs when we eat protein. Protein, being an acidic food, causes the parathyroid to rob our bones and tissues of calcium to restore blood alkalinity. As you may well imagine, this action enhances bone loss. To assist in keeping bone mass, diet should be addressed (since calcium supplements and osteoporosis medications are not effective against this process). In fact, supplemental calcium may lead to other problems, such as claudication. Another situation that naturally creates acidity within the body is the aging process. This imbalance also accompanies conditions like arthritis, inflammation, cancer, respiratory ailments and bone loss, as described above.

Proportion of Daily Acid to Alkaline Foods

If the whole notion of putting appropriate foods together seems too foreign, the following guideline may help: Alkaline (80 percent) is two fruits a day, 6–8 vegetables (several of these could be in a salad), combined with 20 percent acid, or one starch, one protein (or 2–3 small proteins, divided up throughout the day).

Alkaline Foods

Fruits: Most fruits are alkaline, with the few exceptions being berries, like cranberries and citrus fruit. Lemons have an alkaline ash, and are therefore considered alkaline-forming. Research does show that, while citrus is initially acidic when first eaten, it becomes alkaline through the digestive process.

Vegetables: This food group is predominately alkaline. White potatoes are acidic, and corn becomes acid forming 24 hours after being picked.

Grains: Amaranth, millet, wild rice (black grain) and quinoa are alkaline. Because gluten intolerance is a common problem with gut disorders, grains need to be avoided unless you know for a fact that the ones you choose to eat are gluten-free. There are a few that may be tolerated by certain people, such as oats, rice, corn, sorghum and millet.

Beans: Green beans (string), lima beans, peas, soybeans, soy products and snap peas, are alkaline.

Alkalizing Protein: Almonds, chestnuts, millet, tempeh (fermented), tofu (fermented) and whey protein powder are examples of alkaline-forming proteins.

Nuts: The alkaline nuts are almonds, chestnuts, coconut and pine nuts.

Seeds (Sprouted): Alfalfa, broccoli, chia, mung bean, radish and sesame are good alkaline choices.

Sugars: Sweeteners such as brown rice, honey, guava, barley malt, the herb stevia and sucanat are better alternatives to white cane sugar, corn syrup and other commercial sugar additives.

Drinks: Raw alkaline fruit juice, vegetable juices and green juice are superior liquid food sources. Herbal teas are alkaline drinks, and are predominantly caffeine-free.

Dairy: Alkaline dairy products usually contain probiotics (friendly gut flora) like yogurt, kefir, clabbered milk and buttermilk (all unsweetened).

Acid Foods
Protein: Animal meat, fish and fats.

Processed Food: Processed foods in general are acid forming.

Dairy: All dairy products save for the ones listed above are acid forming (this includes cheeses, margarine and butter).

Beverages: Coffee is highly acidic, as is black tea, soda, processed and sweetened juices, wine, alcohol and beer.

Tomato: Cooked sauces and other processed tomato products are acidic.

Fruits: Grapefruit, oranges, cranberries, plums, prunes and blueberries are acidic.

Grains: In general, grains are acidic, with few exceptions. This includes their flour counterparts.

Rice: All forms of rice are acidic.

Legumes and Beans: Black beans, chick peas, kidney beans, lentils, lima beans, pinto beans, red beans and white beans are some examples.

Fats and Oils: Samples of acidic fats and oils include avocado oil, canola oil, corn oil, hemp seed oil, flax oil, lard, olive oil, safflower oil, and sunflower oil.

Cereals: Made from acidic grains as they are, cereals are predominantly acidic.

Nuts: Brazil nuts, cashews, filberts, pecans, peanuts, pistachios, walnuts and macadamia, to name a few, are examples of acid causing nuts.

Seeds: Much the same as other acid nuts, a few examples are pumpkin, sunflower and wheat germ.

Sweeteners: Artificial sugar substitutes are acidic.

Dietary Suggestions for Crohn's Disease, Ulcerative Colitis, and Celiac Disease

Note: This Initial Protocol is always implemented alongside other dietary and supplemental recommendations.

The following dietary instructions have aided in the treatment of many gastrointestinal disorders, such as ulcerative colitis, crohn's disease, celiac disease and chronic diarrhea. An essential element of the diet that must be adhered to, and which is continually repeated, is as follows: no foods containing carbohydrates other than those listed and found in fruits, vegetables, nuts, seeds, honey and yogurt are to be ingested. This is easier said and understood than done. The labeling of foods is often inadequate for those on a precise diet, especially since some ingredients have several names and are not easily recognized as a forbidden item.

Certain fruits and vegetables have laxative properties and must be used with caution when diarrhea is present. Once diarrhea has been remedied, most fruits and vegetables may be eaten (as long as they are being digested). Safe sweeteners include raw honey (in moderation), guava and the herb stevia. Depending on symptoms and tolerance, after a week or two, fruits may be tested, as long as they are ripe, peeled and cooked. Fruits in their raw state should not be added to the diet until diarrhea is under control. The same applies to raw vegetables such as salad greens, carrots and onions.

An Exception to Every Rule

The Good News

With the exception of the patient described in the lengthy case history in Chapter 6 (who was unable to digest carbohydrates and sugars properly), the recommendations I make regarding many of the restricted items have not been a problem for my patients. When it comes to starches and grains, it is my experience that most allowable gluten-free carbohydrates (deemed safe for a celiac diet) have worked for the majority of people. Food items that bother you right now may not once your gut has had a chance to heal. Others, like gluten or corn, can remain an irritant for a much longer period, or even indefinitely. Examples of foods tolerated by most patients include white potatoes, quinoa, rice, amaranth, millet, oats, several beans like red and black (unless gas is a problem), lentils and the pea family. Timing and food preparation are determining factors; make sure to ease into solid food. The same goes for broadening the variety of groceries being purchased.

There have been cases where a food item is considered safe and yet presented a problem. The diet may need to be as individualized as you are; nonetheless, this is not as insurmountable a task as it would seem. When something does not agree with you, your body lets you know quite quickly. Sometimes it can be tricky to decide which item was the culprit, especially if you ate several different foods at one meal. In these cases, remove a few that you feel may be the problem and reintroduce them one at a time.

The Bad News

Your diet can't do it alone.

In treating the many chronic and long-term case histories for gut diseases, simply changing one's diet has not worked in ensuring a full reversal of these gastrointestinal complaints, especially in a timely manner. The diet is a large component, particularly in the initial stages; however, many other symptoms such as diarrhea, bleeding, pain, infection, inflammation, gas, bloating, nausea and others require complementary medicine to replace prescribed medications and to alleviate symptoms. People are used to taking drug medications, and want a quick fix or a magic pill. But impatience is a culprit in and of itself. The body needs time to restore itself and become strong and resistant. Through properly feeding and supporting the body, the process of healing and restoration takes place much more quickly—remarkably so. During this phase, the initial symptoms will fade away along with the medications they originally called for.

What Else is Needed?

The other requirement needed to achieve real, timely healing is to address the many deficiencies and imbalances throughout the body. How limiting the diet has become and the level of malnourishment that has occurred will dictate the start-up program of supplementation. Many nutrients are best found in whole food supplements, such as through juicing, nutritional yeast, chlorophyll, protein powders, vegetable proteins, sea plants and algae and essential fatty acids. Through these and other specific items, all the areas of body can be supported at once. This area of nutrition empowers the body to heal and rebalance itself. The restoration of energy is one the first noticeable improvements, along with a lessening of troublesome symptoms. Several supplements taken at the onset will not be required for a continuance of health, but will rather be for boosting a low functioning area in the body. Be sure to address the endocrine system as a whole as certain glands will require special attention (as has been noted in this book). Other critical areas are the immune system, blood levels of B12 and hemoglobin, nervous system, circulation and your emotional well-being.

When recommending a diet, it is important to emphasize what is *not* to be eaten, rather than what *is*. A food and symptom diary is a must in order to accurately track a person's progress (or lack thereof). Enormous success has been achieved in alleviating the debilitating symptoms of intestinal disorders through restricted dietary suggestions. But discipline on the part of the person doing the cooking, or on the part of the person taking care of themselves, is critical. If allowances are made in such instances—moments of weakness such as having "just a taste" of cake, ice cream or any other forbidden food—recovery time will be seriously delayed. If the dietary program is followed carefully for one month, there should be noticeable improvement. These positive changes will provide the encouragement needed to commit oneself to the long haul.

The Immune System and Brain Connection

Once the commitment has been made, the following recommendations should be followed for approximately two years (or one year after the last symptom has disappeared). This applies to the known triggers or culprits of symptoms such as gluten, chemicals and any allergic substance or food that has shown to be a persistent problem. The body happens to be brilliant; an unwanted food element registers equally as a foreign bacteria. Most people would understand why an antibiotic does not continue to work well (or at all) when it is reintroduced into a body after building up resistance. The immune and brain connection comes into play. The immune system recognizes the bacteria and the brain makes a blueprint of the offender. The next time it shows up, the body immediately recognizes it and sets up its defense mechanisms to remove and destroy the invader. This is the same scenario for any food or substance that finds itself in areas of the body that it should never be in, like having gluten in the blood.

In order to circumvent this, we essentially need to "fake out" the brain. I have noticed that many items, so long as it is not an inherited weakness, can be successfully reintroduced back into the diet after a protracted period of time. The problem I most often see is that when people are feeling better, which oftentimes happens quickly, they test the waters. Again, lack of patience is the culprit. I usually notice this occurrence within a few weeks to a few months, in which strong symptoms show up again. This usually serves to reinforce the discipline required to adhere to an elimination diet.

If any food gives you a severe allergenic reaction, discontinue it at once. If an allowable food does not agree with you, leave it alone for now; perhaps in a week's time, try it again in reduced amounts. It is not uncommon when first starting a new way of eating for the patient to have continued discomfort, usually lasting a week or two. At this time, supplements may be adding to the problem, especially when none have been taken prior. The preparation of food and finding a way to incorporate supplements is critical to ensuring that the body receives adequate nutrition. Mix supplements into yogurt, protein powders, soups, juices and around meals to buffer the stomach lining. In cases such as these, the gastrointestinal tract, including the stomach, needs a bit of time to "calm down" before healing can commence. Think in terms of easy digestible food forms and high quality nutrition—less work and more nourishment for the body.

As previously mentioned, it is advisable to keep a journal of your daily progress. Include the discomfort levels of gas and other symptoms. If you feel significant improvement has not been achieved, the diet may need to be adjusted and a closer look at any nutritional deficiencies. Complementary medicine may also be applied to lessen any unwanted symptoms.

Gluten Alert: FDA Implements New Standards

Research has shown that gluten alone can cause damage to the intestine. This becomes evident in all those who have celiac disease. It is crucial that anyone with gut dysbiosis complaints similar to that of celiac avoid all foods containing wheat, oats, barely and rye.

Along these lines, the FDA recently published a new regulation on August 5, 2013 defining the term *gluten-free* for voluntary food labeling. Margaret A. Hamburg, M.D., the FDA Commissioner, explained that the new labeling regulation will provide a uniform standard definition to help people with celiac disease and other similar diseases in making food choices with confidence.

The gluten-free standard requires that food labeled as *gluten-free* contain less than 20 parts per million of gluten, which the FDA states "is the lowest level that can be consistently detected in foods using valid scientific analytical tools." The statement continues: "Most people with celiac disease can tolerate foods with very small amounts of gluten. This level is consistent with those set by other countries and international bodies that set food safety standards." Until the FDA recently formulated the new rule for products to be labeled *gluten-free*, no such standards or definitions existed federally in the food industry to monitor the labeling of *gluten-free*. The FDA estimated at the time that five percent of foods labeled as *gluten-free* contained 20 parts per million, or more, of gluten protein.

This new definition claim of *gluten-free* was implemented across the food industry. Food manufacturers had one year to bring their labels into compliance with the new requirements. This standardization also required that foods labeled *no gluten*, *free of gluten*, and *without gluten* meet the new definition for *gluten-free*. Hopefully, this action has made it easier for people with gluten intolerances to shop for food.

Unfortunately, the new standard does not affect foods that are not labeled *gluten-free*; therefore, you must check the labels carefully. Foods and ingredients that may contain gluten include the following: cold cuts, soups, soy sauce, candy, hydrolyzed vegetable protein (HVP), hydrolyzed plant protein (HPP), starch, modified food starch, vegetable protein (TVP), binders, fillers, shelf extenders, malt, and natural flavorings.

For more information, check with the Celiac Disease Foundation (www.celiac.org) or the Celiac Sprue Association (www.csaceliacs.org).

Starting the Diet

For severe symptoms of diarrhea, bleeding, malnutrition, chronic fatigue and inflammation, refer to the Initial Quick Start Program in Chapter 5 for more detailed information. The following daily start-up diet may be too hard to digest. Always think of easily digestible foods, with preparation geared towards a consistency that requires less work by the stomach. At this time, incorporate vegetable and green juices, easily digested proteins such as hemp, soy and pea powders in smoothies or drinks, and healing teas. Also, consider nutritious meals in the form of soups, either blended or strained. Upon reintroducing solid food in a more traditional style of meal preparation, do not combine foods—in other words, no meat *and* potatoes (a starch and protein).

When initiating the diet, abdominal pains and diarrhea are usually severe. In such cases, the following diet should be maintained for five days; otherwise, one or two days may be sufficient. There is no limitation as to the quantity eaten.

Juicing and Fiber

Initially, my patients consume vegetable juice and liquid chlorophyll in water in addition to the following diet or other similar eating plans. Most quickly notice the healing effects and a boost in energy. I also suggest extra fiber in the juice to combat diarrhea effects, such as ground flax seeds (1–2 tablespoons), or guar gum (1–2 teaspoons). This form of nutrition speeds up the healing process. If for some reason the juice is unsuitable because of taste or diarrhea, adjust the formula temporarily to taste.

Breakfast Suggestions

- Dry cottage cheese (uncreamed cottage cheese), combined with homemade yogurt for added moisture.
- Eggs, scrambled, boiled or poached.
- Unsweetened pineapple juice or grape juice, diluted with ½ water or freshly made vegetable juice.
- Unflavored gelatin sweetened with juice, or allowed sweetener.

If you cannot find dry cottage cheese, you can replace it with cream cheese made by straining yogurt through gauze or other sterilized cloth for 6–8 hours. Other names for dry cottage cheese are "farmer's cheese" or "baker's cheese." Regardless of its name, characteristics include a dry white curd with no extra fluid added to it. Because of how it is processed, the lactose content is insignificant—approximately 1 percent.

Another good breakfast option would be a smoothie made with yogurt, lactose-free whey powder, ground flax seeds and flax seed oil, and a raw egg yolk. If you are certain that you can tolerate certain fruits, you may add them. To this mixture, add slippery elm and supplements, or anything else that is well tolerated. This can also be consumed as a snack or for lunch, as long as the formula is tolerated.

An additional option for extra support (if needed) is slippery elm powder made into a gruel, using 1–2 tablespoons of slippery elm powder combined with a small amount of hot water, aloe vera gel or juice. You may sweeten it with honey or stevia. Eat by the spoonful and chew slowly. This mixture can be eaten on its own at anytime, and is good for inflammation.

Lunch Choices
Soup Selections

- Homemade veal joint broth or chicken soup with puréed carrots and herbs.
- Pea soup made from red, yellow or green split peas or whole dried peas.
- Vegetable soup with whole or split peas.

Protein Selections

- Broiled fish or minced beef
- Chicken or turkey
- Soybeans products if tolerated
- Black beans or red beans (if gas isn't a real problem; otherwise, delay)

Dessert
- Homemade pumpkin pie (substituting cream with yogurt or blended dry cottage cheese, and replace the brown sugar with honey or stevia)
- Gelatin (if it is homemade)

Dinner: Combinations of above.
You may add cooked fruit, banana and vegetables once the symptoms of diarrhea, gas and cramping have subsided. As you begin to feel better, the

rest of the diet can be introduced (with exception to the cabbage family, which should not be introduced until diarrhea has all but vanished). Other foods may be introduced earlier, depending on the stability of the patient and their progress. Otherwise, substantial improvement is noticed approximately three weeks into the program, which usually continues.

Occasionally, even when following this regimen faithfully, a temporary annoyance may occur in the form of a cold or respiratory infection. There is always a reason as to why you pick up a bacterial infection, even when you are making great progress. One reason is the body eliminating on a cellular level; another is your immune system may continue to be compromised, leaving you vulnerable to germs. I have never found these minor incidences to pose a problem of any significance. As a person's health escalates, so too will their resistance to illness, along with a quicker recovery time.

Recovery Times

Typically, spastic colon and celiac disease may be cured in approximately a year's time. Crohn's disease and ulcerative colitis usually takes two years; although having said that, I notice most patients are living a vastly improved lifestyle within 2–6 months. It is advisable to stay on the diet for a year after the last symptom has disappeared. At this time, forbidden food may be added in small amounts, about one food per week. Assuming the food was tolerated, you may try adding another. If symptoms return, remain on your dietary program. This scenario also applies to sensitive systems, or a very leaky gut that has not adequately healed over. In respect to severe allergies to gluten or other substances, especially in a Type "A" Crohn's individuals and celiac cases, they may need to adhere to certain specifics in their dietary program indefinitely. Remember that your body cannot be coerced into tolerating something just because you now *feel* much better, especially when the culprit is a strongly-inherited weakness or an inability to digest and assimilate properly.

Suggested Foods

The following list of foods is an example of the more easily digested foods (which should be eaten), and those not usually tolerated when on a restrictive or healing diet.

Avoid: Spicy foods, greasy and fried foods, pepper, caffeine, alcohol, tobacco, chocolate, carbonated beverages, margarine, all refined sugar and flour products, all processed meat (including lunchmeat), hotdogs, smoked meat/fish or breaded meat/fish and chemical additives for seasoning or preservatives.

Note: Typically, processed meats contain starch, lactose or sucrose and whey powder.

Grain Type Foods

Best Grains When Gluten- or Carbohydrate-Sensitive
- Quinoa
- Wild and black rice
- Montina rice
- Wild rice pasta or Montina rice grass
- Grain substitutes may be tried with caution, such as teff flour, adzuki bean flour, chia flour, chickpea and fava flour.

Refer to Chapter 13 for a list of additional gluten-free flours and thickening agents.

Prohibited Grains and Flours: Depending on the disorder and tolerance of the individual, the following grains (and those which are similar in composition) would be temporarily or permanently removed. Symptoms and conditions will dictate the outcome and duration of an eliminative diet. For example, if a person had type "A" Crohn's disease, they would permanently leave most starches and sugars out of their daily diet plan, concentrating on vegetables, proteins and some fruits.

For a much longer list, refer to the list of gluten-free grains, flours, ingredients and foods in Chapter 13.

Grains and Flours Not Acceptable for a Type "A" Crohn's Patient

Amaranth	Faba	Soybeans
Barley	Garbanzo	Triticale
Bean sprouts	Millet	Wheat
Buckwheat	Mungbeans	Wheatgerm
Bulgur	Oats	Grain substitutes,
Chickpeas	Rice	such as
Corn	Rye	cottonseed
Couscous	Spelt	

Many of these choices that are gluten and corn-free have been tolerated even by patients with severe gut dysbiosis complaints. Refer to Chapter 13 for a list of other related items from wheat sources.

> Seaweed is a very healthy complement to our diets. It comes in various forms that can be tolerated and helpful. Sea plants like seaweed are one of the few sources of iodine, which is required to enable the thyroid to produce thyroid hormone. Seaweed may be purchased in supplement form

Dairy Products

All alkaline dairy is highly recommended as part of a healthy diet, but in the case of lactose intolerance, non-dairy forms must be purchased. Coconut and almond milk may also be tried. Acidophilus and bifidus culture (probiotics) is readily available in health food stores, as well as many grocery stores.

Otherwise, avoid buttermilk, yogurt, sour cream, dried milk solids or liquid milk of any type. Note that it is possible to purchase sour cream which contains virtually no lactose. Only occasionally do I see a patient unable to tolerate commercial acidophilus and bifidus supplements.

Cheeses Not Permitted

Cream cheese	Mozzarella
Cottage cheese	Neufchatel
Feta, Greek or other	Primmest
(may try after 6 months)	Processed cheese or spreads
Gjetost	Ricotta cheese
Gruyere	Tofutti cheese

Cheeses Allowed With Caution

Initially, I recommend all dairy sourced cheese to be omitted until sufficient healing has taken place.

Asiago	Colby
Blue	Dry curd cottage cheese
Brick	Edam
Brie	Gorgonzola
Camembert	Gouda
Cheddar	Gruyere

Havarti
Limburger
Manchego
Monterey jack
Muenster
Oka
Parmesan

Port du Salut
Provolone
Romano
Roquefort
Stilton
Swiss

Proteins

Proteins Permitted

Fresh or frozen lamb
Pork
Chicken
Beef
Fish (canned fish in oil or water)
Homemade yogurt

Eggs
Natural cheeses
Legume family (with caution)
Other gluten-free vegetable
    sourced proteins

Vegetables

Vegetables Permitted

Mainly non-acidic fresh
    vegetables
Lettuce (all varieties)
Dried white navy beans
Adzuki beans
Black beans
Artichoke
Asparagus
Beets
Bok choy
Broccoli
Brussels sprouts
Cabbage
Carrots
Cauliflower
Celery
Chickpeas

Cucumbers
Eggplant
Garlic
Kale
Lentils
Lima beans
Mushrooms
Onions
Parsley
Peas
Peppers
Pumpkin
Split peas
Spinach
Sprouts
Squash
String beans

Sweet potatoes
Tomatoes
Turnips
Watercress

Zucchini
Raw vegetables (suitable as long
   as diarrhea is not active; try
   juicing)

Fruits

Fruits Permitted

Fruits are to be eaten with no added sugar, consumed fresh, raw, cooked or frozen. For sweetening fruits, use raw honey, guava or the herb stevia—no other artificial sweetener.

Acai
Apples
Aronia berries
Apricots
Avocados
Ripe bananas
Cherries
Dragon fruit
Dates (loose, not stuck together
   with sugar or syrup coating)
*Grapefruit
Grapes
Kiwi
Kumquats
Lemons
Limes
Logan berries

Lychee fruit
Mangoes
Melons
Nectarines
*Oranges
Papayas
Peaches
Pears
Persimmons
Pineapples
Prunes
Raisins (dark)
Rhubarb
Tangerines
Wolfberry
All kinds of berries
Fresh coconut and its milk

Initially, these fruits may not be tolerated for being too acidic.

Note: Although oranges and grapefruits are permitted, I recommend avoidance unless they are tree-ripened. Citrus fruit, when transported to areas where they are not natively grown, are unripe when picked and contain a non-beneficial green citric acid. Rhubarb and cranberries should be seldom eaten, for they are high in oxalic acid.

Nuts

Nuts Permitted (With or Without Shells)
*Initially, all nuts and seeds unless in the form of butter or finely ground should be avoided until all symptoms have stabilized.

> Almonds
>
> Brazil nuts
>
> Chestnuts
>
> Hazelnuts
>
> Peanut butter (without additives or roasted in shell may be added with caution)
>
> Pecans
>
> Pint nuts
>
> Unroasted cashews
>
> Walnuts

Nut and Seed Butters: Almond, cashew and hemp are quality choices as long as they digest well.

Other Dietary Restrictions

Vinegar: Only apple cider and white vingar varieties are permitted (gourmet vinegars have added sugar). The concern lies with the use of raw materials such as barley, malt and other malt grains to make vinegar. Therefore, individuals with gluten intolerance (like celiac cases) may safely consume distilled white vinegar or products that may contain it. Condiments such as dill pickles and olives are permitted, provided they are devoid of sugar. Vinegars with higher sugar content like balsamic are allowed back into the diet only when sufficient healing has taken place.

Pasta: Varieties such as spaghetti and macaroni are not permitted. Substitute with spaghetti squash or julienne zucchini. Gluten-free pasta and noodles are often well tolerated.

Pizza Crusts: Pizza crusts can be made from nut flour, egg, vegetables (such as zucchini), and a permitted cheese combination.

Gluten-Free Crust: Made using 1 cup approved flour mix, 1 tablespoon sugar, 1 teaspoon of baking powder substitute or traditional baking powder, ½ cup milk, ¼ cup potato flour, 1 teaspoon salt, 1 large egg, and 1/8 cup olive oil. Combine together and bake in a 350°F oven for 25 minutes. Add toppings and return to oven.

Baking Powder (Grain-Free): Replace 3 teaspoons of baking powder with 1.5 teaspoons of cream of tarter combined with about 1 teaspoon of baking soda.

Bean and Nut Flours (For Cooking or Baking): When purchasing beans, inquire as to whether they have previously been soaked before being ground; otherwise, soak, cook and purée your favorite variety, to be added to cake recipes (in order to cut down the quantity of nut flour). Use lentil or bean flour sparingly to ensure tolerance. Refer to Chapter 13 for gluten-free grains and flours from bean and nut flours.

Sweets: Do not use products containing refined sugar. This includes many commercial products. Avoid labels with fructose, sucrose, dextrose or corn syrup. Avoid molasses, corn syrup, and maple syrup. Note that a person is not totally denied sweets on this diet; your favorite cakes or cookies can instead be made with honey, stevia (herb), guava, dried fruits (sparingly), and nuts and seeds (when sufficient healing has occurred).

Oils: Grains are not permitted, although cooking and salad oils are allowed when made from grains. You may use corn, soybean, sunflower, and safflower oils. Olive oil is highly endorsed. Use omega 3 oils in dressings such as walnut, almond, flax seed, hemp or chia oil.

Butter: Butter is the spread of choice, not margarine.

Thickening Agents: Thickening agents are not allowed, including the following: cornstarch, arrowroot, tapioca starch or any other starch. This suggestion applies to people who have problems digesting carbohydrates and sugars. For those on a carbohydrate-restricted diet, I have found that guar gum, tapioca, potato starch, rice starch and pectin can be exceptions to this rule. Refer to Chapter 13 for a list of gluten-free ingredients, foods and gluten-free fibers for more cooking ingredient choices.

Common Replacements

Replacing Flour as a Thickener
Items such as corn starch, arrowroot and potato starch have twice the thickening agent potential as flour; therefore, use about half the amount called for first, and then add a bit more if needed. Too much thickening compound can affect the end result of your dish. This is especially true when making sauces and gravies.

Corn Syrup Replacement
Recipes calling for liquid sugar are not interchangeable with granulated versions. For a healthy choice, try agave syrup, or else use another form of sugar and adjust the liquids in the recipe. Honey and molasses can work; however, the taste will be quite different, depending on the recipe, and for this reason may not be compatible.

Gravy: Thicken with cooked vegetables like onions.

Maltol: Despite its name, maltol is safe for gluten-intolerant diets. Maltol is a derivative of the bark of larch trees, pine needles, chicory and roasted malt. It is used as a flavoring agent to produce the wonderful odor found in freshly baked products.

Caramel: Caramel, made from sugar molecules, is used for its coloring aspects and taste. It does not possess gluten and is thereby safe for celiac and other gluten-sensitive individuals.

Monosodium Glutamate (MSG): MSG is the sodium salt of glutamic acid, an amino acid found in many foods. In the past, it had been produced from both wheat gluten and sugar beet molasses. But today, MSG is being produced almost entirely from sugar beet molasses in a highly purified form. Because of this change in manufacturing, most authorities agree that it is now harmless. Therefore, celiac and other gluten-intolerant people should not be concerned about the use of foods containing MSG.

Caution: Since 2009, wheat-derived MSG has been found in products imported from Asia. R5 ELISA testing is needed to confirm its suitability in the gluten-free diet.

Condiments: Check condiments (like ketchup) very carefully for their ingredients. These types of items are usually very high in sugar, and may contain gluten. Gourmet mustards, for example, have many additives which must be avoided; use plain mustard instead.

Bouillon Cubes: Bouillon cubes and instant soup bases, used to enhance flavor, are not recommended. Check with whole foods and health stores for more suitable choices.

Beverages and Liquids

Grape Juice: Light or dark grape juice is a good choice; avoid frozen juice unless you can find one that has not been sweetened.

Pineapple Juice: A healthy choice, pineapple is a product without sugar, and it may be canned, frozen or fresh.

Fresh Juice: Fresh juices of allowed fruits and vegetables are highly recommended and very beneficial. Green juices are concentrated powerhouses of nutrition. Suggestions include juiced kale, spinach, dandelion, grasses and sprouts. You may sweeten if you desire, and the use of fresh lemon juice can cut the bitter taste. Avoid orange juice and grapefruit juice in the morning, if diarrhea is active. These fruits can promote symptoms of loose stools or diarrhea even in people *without* a gut disorder.

Milk Substitutes: Currently, there are a number of alternative milk substitutes available, such as soy, rice, potato and oat milks. Nut-derivative milks include almond, cashew and coconut. When replacing dairy milk with a non-dairy substitution, substitute in a ratio of 1:1. Caution should be employed when introducing tree nut milk products to anyone with a nut allergy.

Evaporated Milk: Evaporated milk contains 60 percent less water. Choose a milk substitute such as soy or rice and simmer until it has been reduced by 60 percent. Be careful not to burn or scald the milk. Another alternative for evaporated milk is to substitute coconut milk (in a ratio of 1:1) in the recipe; however, the recipe will have a slight coconut flavor and is thus not suited for all recipes.

Tea: Black tea is acceptable, when brewed very weak.

Herbal Teas: Herbal teas are safe as long as they do not have a laxative effect. Most herbal teas are welcomed, especially those that will soothe and promote healing. Nervine teas for calming are great as well; for example, lemon balm, chamomile, St. John's wort, passionflower, and valerian will help with sleeplessness and stress.

Smoothies and Shakes: Smoothies and shakes can be made with home-made yogurt, allowed whey powder, hemp powder, pea powder, rice bran powder and fruit, sweetened with raw honey or the herb stevia.

Coffee Substitutes: Subsituting for coffee is a good choice; ground chicory is a great alternative.

Very Dry Wine (White or Red): Very dry wine is allowed, in both white and red varieities. If a sweeter taste is desired, add a crushed saccharin tablet, stevia or a little honey. On occasion, rye, gin, scotch, bourbon, vodka and other liquors are permitted, but not recommended. Sherry, cordials, brandy and liqueurs are *not* allowed. Club soda is permitted as a mixer. Wine is derived from grapes, and is therefore allowed. Wines that fall under the heading as being fortified, such as sherry or port, contain additional alcohol—they are also approved.

Alcohol and Beer: Alcohol and beer are *not* permitted. Besides the issues involving the original source material used to make these beverages (which are of a concern similar to vinegar) the use of alcohol and beer is prohibited under the initial recommendation that patients stop breaking their bodies down. Even once a patient has made significant progress, I would only consider including certain irritating substances in their diet. Beer is made from barley and may contain 1–2 mg of prolamins per pint (570 ml). Distilled alcoholic beverages such as gin, vodka, scotch whisky and rye whiskey are made from wheat, barley or rye. Since they are distilled, they do not contain prolamins, and may not present a problem. Investigate to be sure before consuming.

Apple Juice: Apple juice has become a problem, as many manufacturers mislabel their products. Many times, sugar or corn syrup has been added without being declared. Health food stores and the health section in many local grocery stores are particularly good sources of juice products. Juice boxes may present a problem, even when no sugar is listed on its labeling. Many people have expressed that these juices are not well tolerated.

Coffee: Coffee is far too acidic to digest, and should be completely removed from our diets. The properties in the bean are harmful to our beneficial gut flora.

V-8 and Canned Tomato Juice: Tomato juice can replace tomato sauces and paste for cooking, though my preference would be to make your own using a juicer. Note that these are not always tolerated, especially when inflammation is a problem. Make certain to check for salt content.

Diet Soft Drinks: These beverages may contain lactose if they are sweetened with aspartame or Nutri-Sweet; for this reason, it's best to avoid them. If no other choices are available, one per week is permitted. Diet soft drinks with saccharin are permitted 2-3 times a week, if so desired. Avoid all other soda choices, as they are extremely high in sugar. Note that while in many cases these drinks may be tolerated, professionally I do not recommend any of my patients drink chemical-laden beverages such as soda while on my program.

Other Beverages: Beverages that seem similar to the following: soybean milk, instant tea or coffee, postum, enzyme treated milk or coffee substitutes (which usually contain malt) are to be avoided. Also, avoid tomato juice combinations such as Clamato. Additionally, soda, energy drinks, or commercial fruit juice and vitamin drinks (as well as any similar products) should be removed from the diet.

Agar-Agar or Carrageenan: Carrageenan (a compound extracted from red seaweed) and agar-agar are used by the food industry as a stabilizing and suspending agent, for a variety of functions, and should be *avoided*. Due to carrageenan's ability to stabilize milk proteins, it is widely used in milk and chocolate milk products such as ice cream, cottage cheese, milk chocolate and so forth.

Medications: Several medications have added sugar such as sucrose and lactose. Ask your pharmacist to suggest a brand without these sugars.

Gum: Be aware that gum is often coated with flour, which contains gluten.

Example of a Daily Menu Once Sufficient Healing has Taken Place

Breakfast
- ½ cup plain yogurt (eaten first; a little raw honey may be added)
- Millet or amaranth grain (cooked cereal)
- Milk or dairy replacement
- Herbal tea

Lunch
- Salmon or tuna salad made with homemade mayonnaise, garnished with lettuce and tomato (or homemade squash or split pea soup)
- Date loaf
- Perrier, club soda, or fruit juice (alone or combined)

Lunch Choice #2
- Lentil and wild rice pilaf mixed with sautéed vegetables
- Homemade gelatin
- Herbal tea
- Puréed soup of tolerated vegetables and protein (as a substitute for pilaf above)

Afternoon Snack (Around 3:00 PM)
- Vegetable cocktail

Dinner
- Asparagus and tomato salad with homemade vinaigrette dressing
- Spaghetti (made with spaghetti squash or thinly sliced zucchini) combined with ground beef or chicken, herbs, garlic, olive oil and tomato juice.
- Sauce option: In a blender, place fresh tomatoes with their skins and seeds removed. Add olive oil, 1 garlic clove, parsley and a small amount of sweet onion (or 1 shallot). Add 1 teaspoon of raw honey and any other herbs, to taste. Blend and add immediately to hot pasta of your choice.
- Tofu (if tolerated) may substitute for the protein

Dessert
- Strawberry mousse made with yogurt, eggs, honey, unflavored gelatin and strawberries

Tea
- Any allowable teas, including herbal teas

Treatment Plan for Colitis (Microscopic, Collagenous, and Lymphocytic Colitis)

The terms colitis and inflammatory bowel disease, which describe Crohn's disease and pancolitis, are fast becoming household words. Collagenous colitis and its various referents fall under a similar guideline, given its variation on its colitis-like symptoms.

The symptoms of microscopic colitis could also be a precursor to its more undesirable relatives—pancolitis and IBD—especially if left untreated or unsuccessfully treated. The condition of collagenous colitis was first identified in Sweden, along with its subset of lymphocytic colitis, which has many symptoms in common. Both have been grouped under the umbrella of microscopic colitis.

Symptoms

The main complaint with microscopic colitis is watery diarrhea and too-frequent bowel movements, both of which may be accompanied by abdominal cramping and pain. Fatigue is a common companion to these conditions, especially when they are chronic or too frequent. The loss of electrolytes and nutrition is a major concern with any prolonged symptoms of diarrhea. The immune system will weaken, as will the body's ability to repair itself and function appropriately.

Causes

Typically, the related causes for collagenous colitis appear to be atypical among middle-aged women and those who live in the industrialized areas of the world. Prolonged usage of medications, especially those for pain and inflammation, or bad diet habits coupled with NSAIDs and pain medications seem to top the list when comparing case histories. There may also be other causes similar to those associated with the more severe gastrointestinal complaints involving autoimmune disorders, food antigens and food poisoning.

The following list of drugs has been implicated and incriminated as a cause for microscopic colitis:[11] proton pump inhibitors (PPIs), including Iansoprazole (Prevacid, Prevacid SoluTab), Esomeprazole (Nexium) and Omeprazole (Prilosec, Zegerid). Additionally, the Statin Simvastatin (Zocor); H2 Blocker Ranitidine (Zantac); P2Y12 Inhibitor Ticolpidine (Tilcid) and SSRI Sertraline (Zoloft) should be considered as part of this list.

Treatment Protocol
A foreboding sense of danger is not uncommon when symptoms of collagenous colitis persist. This feeling of not being safe can expedite symptoms of loose stools and bouts of diarrhea. As with IBS symptoms, emotions play a major role in lessening symptoms (especially in the beginning of treatment) until the bouts of diarrhea and frequent bowel movements subside. Once there is noticeable improvement, a person will not focus as much on what might be; this in and of itself will alleviate the associated emotions of anxiety which ultimately hasten—and may well ensure—the feared outcome.

Supplement
Start with a few supplements and the initial diet protocol. Many times, this alone will work, unless the body is fatigued and without the energy needed for repair and rebuilding, or if you are missing too many of nutrients normally required for a healthy functioning immune system. In such cases, build the body up more quickly using raw vegetable and green juices. Include supplements (a standard requirement for health maintenance) such as omega 3 fatty acids (found in fish and flax seed oils), zinc, magnesium, B vitamins, and vitamins A, D, C and E. Many nutrients will be picked up through the vegetable juice formula. Information about raw juices and supplementation can be referenced throughout this book for further guidance.

You can also consider including liquid chlorophyll, a concentrated green juice that is loaded with minerals and directly increases the hem portion of the blood matrix. Chlorophyll's alkalizing capabilities are extremely valuable for diarrhea, and enhance nutrition. For a liquid concentrate version,

---

11 Based on studies involving subjects who took anti-inflammatory NSAIDs for six months or longer, and who determined the drug to be the source of their microscopic colitis symptoms. Upon finishing the study and no longer taking NSAIDs, some subject's symptoms of diarrhea improved.

add 2 teaspoons to a cup of water; or, if the product suggests concentrated drops, take 15 drops or ¼ teaspoon three times a day in water. Sip often throughout the day.

Fiber May Be Necessary

For quicker success when combating symptoms of diarrhea, fiber is a necessary component. The integration of fiber is symptom-specific; the more persistent your symptoms, the more often fiber will be needed during the day. Fiber will slow down the elimination process and allow for more assimilation of nutrients. Incorporate finely ground flax seeds (2 tablespoons) in water just before you eat, and in liquid between meals. Add to the mixture any supplements normally taken during this time. Additional fiber can also be mixed into vegetable juice, smoothies or protein drinks. The goal is to see a formed stool; it is for this reason that fiber may need to be taken between meals, as well as during. For chronic or severe symptoms of diarrhea, this could mean six times a day or more until improvement is noticed. It is a quick process; simply have a quantity of fiber with you or at work and take it often for a desired result, reducing as symptoms decrease. The goal is to see how well-formed your stool becomes with just fiber. If the fecal matter becomes too firm, simply cut back on your fiber intake.

Probiotics and Anti-Viral and Anti-Bacterial Tinctures

When looking to include a quality probiotic product in your diet, first take as directed by your brand of choice. Purchase an anti-viral or anti-bacterial formula as a tincture from a health store and take 10 drops six times a day. Continue for five days and assess your improvement. If progress is noticeable, reduce tincture dosage to three times a day for another five days. Along with this protocol, you must avoid irritants to the stomach and intestinal tract. If symptoms continue to be manageable and improve, reduce tincture formulas to 5 drops three times a day for another five days. After this point, stop tincture formulas and continue feeding your body well with necessary supplements and highly nutritious food that are easily digested. Do not be in a hurry to add coffee back into your daily diet; it is too acidic and irritating.

If Diarrhea Persists

By avoiding the restricted items in your diet, you are enhancing your ability to heal faster. Many of these suggestions will be temporary; for example, the number of dietary restrictions and certain remedies like anti-viral tinctures and extra fiber are not permanent fixtures to your intake. To reiterate, avoid coffee, black tea, soda, alcohol, nuts and seeds (unless in butter form), salt and refined sugar, dairy (such as milk and cheese), processed food, all junk foods, hard-to-digest foods (like large portions of animal protein); also, do not eat meat and starch together in a single sitting (such as meat and potatoes); this food combining greatly reduces the efficacy of your digestive enzymes.

However, if you notice that your symptoms persist even while following this protocol carefully, then you must look at the possibility of food intolerances such as gluten, dairy and the chemicals in foods and food items. You would then need to incorporate suggested protocols for the symptoms of colitis or IBD disorders. A closer look at deficiencies or nutrients that are needed by your body, along with complementary medicine to treat your symptoms of diarrhea, nausea, pain, fatigue, and nervousness and stress, may well be necessary.

Check out the Initial Protocol and the Quick Start Program in this book for additional help and choices when dealing with the symptoms of diarrhea and boosting the body. Additionally, replacements for antibiotics, pain medication, inflammation, nausea, gas, bloating and anxiety medications are all referenced in this book.

Treatment Plan and Diet for Irritable Bowel Syndrome (IBS)

As with other gut complaints, IBS involves a number of factors that compromise the immune system and the body's delicate balance. Stress is one such example, which affects not only the major systems in our body but disrupts the intricate balance of our intestinal bacteria. Vast improvement can be achieved with dietary and lifestyle changes for those who suffer from irritable bowel syndrome. In spite of this, there may be a recurring symptom or two which linger on as a constant source of aggravation. IBS is unpredictable, and there is no magical cure or quick treatment for this disorder. The goal of treating IBS, in order of importance, is stable and regular bowel movements and relief from abdominal pain. Pain may be associated with inflammation. Once bowel movements become more consistent (neither too hard nor too soft), abdominal pain is often relieved. Symptoms such as bloating and gas will also improve with reliable, regular bowel movements. When constipation is not a factor, bloating and pain are lessened, and sometimes relieved with bowel evacuation.

Suggested Causes and Factors

Continuing from the overview in Chapter 3, the incidence of IBS can comprise many variables.

In discovering the one or several causes of irritable bowel syndrome, we must investigate many options. Again, these may include *one* or *several* of the following points:

- Parasites, or the overgrowth of bacteria, candida and fungus
- Food sensitivities and allergies (always high on the list)
- Anxiety, emotional issues or stress
- Alcohol, coffee, tea, cigarettes and recreational drugs
- Excess sugar, including hidden sugars such as corn syrup (which is being added to almost everything)
- Citrus fruits, such as oranges, grapefruit or limes (lemons have an alkaline ash and may be tolerable)
- Fats and/or fat allergy
- Chemical sensitivities
- Inadequate fiber
- Nutrient deficiencies and poor diet
- Repeated use of antibiotics or other medications that may have caused inflammation
- Prolonged usage of medications
- Digestion difficulties and eating hastily
- Eating at irregular times or a diet too high in processed foods

As with other intestinal disorders, a bland diet is recommended during flare-ups. You may use a blender or food processor for vegetables and fruits, or use a baby food diet. Both are recommended, as neither have preservatives or salt added. When on a soft diet, include fiber and additional protein sources (such as protein powders) incorporated into nutritional drinks and smoothies.

Certain foods stimulate the secretion of mucus, thereby preventing the absorption of nutrients. Avoid animal fats, margarine, sugar (including derivatives or substitutes), all dairy products with exception to probiotics, spicy foods, fried foods, wheat products and wheat bran, seeds, nuts, all "junk foods" and carbonated beverages. Refrain from smoking and drinking alcohol and coffee, for these substances aggravate the lining of the stomach, intestine and colon.

How to Incorporate Fiber
By simply incorporating easily digestible fiber into your daily routine, you can greatly enhance your ability to regain self control, and in more ways than one. Fiber will add bulk to your stool, making a hard stool softer or a soft stool firmer. When taking fiber supplements, be sure to combine them with your meals, and not just take them before bedtime or away from food. Fiber should be digested with your meals to ensure a consistent, moist and bulky stool.

Ground flaxseeds, psyllium seeds or husks and alfalfa tablets are excellent fiber supplements. These seeds, among others and seed oils, contain vitamin F, which is used to rebuild the mucous lining, especially in the bowel. For other fiber choices, refer to Chapters 5 and 13.

Magnesium Helps
The mineral magnesium, also known as the "relaxer," serves the bowel and body by performing many functions. This all-important element is necessary for effective bowel movements and has been shown to be deficient in people who have damaged intestinal tracts. Magnesium, when found in our food, gives us the greatest benefit. Magnesium is found adequately in our salad vegetables but most abundantly in yellow corn meal. Yellow corn meal is a wonderful laxative and considered to be one of the great bowel toners. Eating yellow corn meal cereal two mornings a week is believed to be beneficial by professionals. Refer to Chapter 10 for more reasons to consider magnesium. However, corn is a common allergen, so include it in your diet with caution.

Aloe Vera Juice
Aloe vera facilitates healing by keeping the colon walls clean of excess mucus and by decelerating adverse food effects. Consume ¼–½ cup, three times daily on an empty stomach. It may also be taken with a colon cleanser which includes gentle herbs to assist digestion and fiber for bulking. An example would be very finely ground flax seeds or psyllium husk powder mixed with herbs like fenugreek powder and licorice root powder. Take 20–30 minutes before a meal.

Nausea
Ginger root (in capsules or tea form) is used to treat nausea associated with an upset stomach. Fresh ginger tea mixed with raw honey is an

excellent choice for an upset stomach and gut. Ginger also has anti-bacterial properties.

Alternatively, add 1 teaspoon of liquid chlorophyll to a cup of water and drink whenever there are symptoms of gas, nausea or pain associated with any gut disorder.

Daily Suggestions for IBS

The following is a general and condensed diet guideline with supplement suggestions, coupled with symptoms. Determine any foods that could create a discomfort in your body. They may not all be allergens, and may rather be temporary sensitivities and intolerances. Unless the offender is a known allergen or inherited weakness, you may reintroduce them slowly, one at a time, all the while logging any symptoms that show up. The goal is to avoid triggering an immune response.

Once the intestinal tract has had sufficient time to heal, the body will typically not respond in the same manner. For example, proteins such as gluten will no longer pass through holes in the gut and into the blood, where they do not belong. When this event is no longer taking place, the immune response will dampen and be less reactive to foreign material.

Diet Guideline for IBS

- Avoid all of the following items: alcohol, coffee, black tea, corn, wheat, citrus, dairy products, processed food and wheat bran. These substances may lead to allergies and adverse symptoms.
- Avoid all sugar forms: fructose corn syrup is inexpensive and an easy way to make food taste better, and so is added to everything. Read labels carefully.
- Increase dietary fiber: ground flax seeds, oat bran, legumes, apple pectin, apples, fruit and vegetables. Examples include 1–2 tablespoons of ground flax seeds added to a pint of buttermilk, kefir or natural yogurt for breakfast. You may add raw honey and fruit, so long as it does not trigger unwanted symptoms.
  - ◆ Note: Even though this form of dairy is alkaline and contains probiotics, these substances must be tolerated first to be included; otherwise, avoid them.

- Acidophilus and Bifidus supplements: Bio-K (fresh half-tub in the morning and the end of day); or probiotic capsules (3–4 a day). Purchase non-dairy varieties if intolerant.
- Liquid whey: throughout the day, take spoonfuls of whey to aid in restoration of intestinal flora and build stomach lining. Check for non-dairy varieties if intolerant.
    - Whey contains one of the highest instances of organic sodium not related to table salt. This mineral is the main element in our lymph system, which is the avenue that feeds our joints, ligaments, synovial fluid and connective tissues. Organic sodium keeps calcium in solution. When calcium is out of solution, it begins the development of such conditions as osteoarthritis (which is primarily a mineral imbalance).

Suggested Supplements for IBS

- Lots of purified water
- Magnesium: liquid or tablet, 500 mg, twice daily.
- Vitamin A: 25000 IU daily
    Raw carrot juice is a rich source of beta-carotene, with carrot juice being my preference. A highly nourishing food source, as opposed to supplemental Vitamin A on its own.
- Aloe vera juice: 2 tablespoons twice daily or (as suggested earlier in this section).
- Liquid chlorophyll: 1–2 teaspoons in water, three times a day or as needed. Very alkalizing and nourishing to the body.
    ◆ Chlorophyll raises the body's red blood count, and is wonderful for anemia.
- Vitamin C, Ester form: 1000–3000 mg daily, or a quality vitamin C in a gel capsule
- Grapefruit extract and/or garlic: 1–3 times a day.
- Apple cider vinegar: 1 teaspoon with meals to aid digestive enzymes.
    ◆ More frequent apple cider vinegar dosages in water will improve and remove mucus and catarrhal conditions.
- Papaya tablets: To help digest protein, take as needed.
- A digestive enzyme supplement that includes the pancreatic enzyme. Consume with each meal, especially when food combining (starch and protein in one meal). Take as needed.

- Ginger: use for cooking and flavoring, or as a tea with honey; very healing.
- Chamomile tea: good for nausea and promotes relaxation.

Herbal Recommendations for IBS
- For diarrhea-related symptoms, refer to Chapters 5 and 11 for remedies.
- Peppermint oil capsules: Use enteric coated capsules, which will pass the stomach and remain intact to reach the intestines, for relief from gas and bowel contractions. Take 1 gel capsule 1–3 times a day or as needed, depending on symptoms of gas and bloating.
- Slippery elm powder: 1 teaspoon per cup of water using the decoction process. 1 cup, 3–5 times a day until relief is felt.
- Comfrey leaf: 1 teaspoon per cup of boiling water using the infusion process. 1 cup, three times a day.
  - Slippery elm and comfrey leaf may be combined and drank together once they have been properly made. When combined, drink 1 cup three times a day.
- Oregano oil or peppermint oil: Add 1 drop of oil in half a cup of water once a day to help control candida overgrowth.
- Parasites and fungus: black walnut hulls extract, caprylic acid, wormwood, goldenseal and cloves may be combined for cleansing either of these pathogens. Take over four weeks as directed by the manufacturer. This group will also target candidia, worms, viruses and bacteria.
- Emotional stress and anxiety. Refer to Chapter 8 for herbal remedies and solutions.

Constipation Recommendations and Solutions

Constipation is a common occurrence, and is not necessarily due to a disease. It is a condition of the bowels marked by suppressed or difficult evacuation. Unfortunately, this situation has become an accepted part of living. To treat constipation, one must first evaluate one's diet and eliminate all known possible causes. The body eliminates systematically for natural reasons. Once we have eaten our food and obtained our energy from it, we have a by-product which needs to be removed from the body. If this waste is not removed from the body within 24 hours, a toxic build-up occurs. The normal transit time for waste is within 18–24 hours. Constipation promotes toxicity build-up, and opens up an invitation for parasitic and microbial infestation. Parasites in both animals and plants are native to all foods and water, with an incubation period of about 36 hours. In reality, the average elimination time of fecal matter is 96 hours; knowing that the body should eliminate solid waste within much shorter time duration, this is problematic to the bearer.

To enhance bowel transit time, incorporate the following suggestions: Drink 6–8 glasses of fluid per day. Eat several fruits and vegetables a day, with additional grains and seeds. When integrating high-fiber foods to be used for increasing bulk, a typical recommendation is half a cup of high fiber cereal, increasing to one and a half cups over several weeks. I prefer cooked cereal for those who are permitted to eat such grains. Include fiber more than once a day, depending on the severity of the condition.

Corn bran is more effective than wheat bran, although it is important to watch for corn, as it is a known allergen. Oat bran may be less irritating. Most forms of fiber have the added benefit of absorbing fat and sugars when incorporated into a meal.

Lowering Cholesterol and Weight Gain

Fiber will lower cholesterol and calories, removing fat by adding water soluble fiber, such as those in the legume family, via the gut. By incorporating this form of fiber at mealtime, you prevent the reabsorption of fat back through the intestines. Fiber also slows down the absorption of sugar, preventing sugar levels from spiking needlessly.

Laxative Herbs and Enemas

It is always far better to have your body functioning on its own power. By adding any laxative-type stimulant to your diet on a consistent basis, you run the risk of causing the colon to become lazy and sluggish. Ideally, you want the colon to have strong muscular layers, to be better able to move fecal matter along under its own power.

Take one tablespoon of flaxseed oil at bedtime. It acts as a stool softener. This is very helpful for hard stools. Flaxseed oil may be taken in the morning, as well for more chronic constipation.

Timing is everything when constipation is a challenge. Some individuals have inherited a lazy colon, which means they will always have to be vigilant on what and when they eat. This type of problem is manageable, but cannot be ignored. For cases such as this one, I also recommend two tablespoons of ground flaxseeds in water, to be consumed before each and every meal. I also recommend adding any supplements into your mixture at this time. Many supplements come in capsules which can be opened, or else in liquid form.

As many of us know, it is not recommended to drink any liquids during a meal. If you are *not* putting salt on your food, you will *not* be thirsty during a meal. If you drink wine with a meal, you will retain calories. It slows the metabolism down and you will not burn fat or calories in the same way. Just imagine how relaxed you feel–everything is slowing down to a crawl!

Why an Enema?

Before I continue with herbal recommendations, I wish to describe a common complication. When the intestinal tract is very impacted and stagnates, adding a stimulant (laxative) will create a lot of gas which, as many people have experienced, is very painful. Laxative herbs like over the counter medications can irritate the system, causing a series of reactions in the body: extra fluid is sent to the gut area, involuntary muscle action is enhanced and gases start to build up, having no place to go because the colon is so backed up. The symptoms that ensue can involve pain and enormous bloating in the abdomen. For this reason, I recommend an enema first to help create room and movement to lessen these symptoms. The gas can then more easily escape and all other symptoms will be relieved. When applying an enema therapy, you may need to do 1–3 in a row in order to create adequate benefit.

The disposable enemas that you purchase from the drug store are much easier to use than the bulb type that is also retailed in these stores. You may reuse the fluid enema container from the box (clean after each use). Refill it with salt and water, strained flaxseed tea or herbs like chamomile or black coffee (remember how irritating coffee is to the colon). This is an effective alternative when away on a holiday and there are no commercial enemas available.

An enema is preferable so long as it is not abused with a colonic or similar procedure that extends far up into the large colon. This procedure is performed at times for medical and health practices, such as accompanying a liver/gallbladder cleanse or a medical test. A procedure such as this one should not become a routine.

Herbal Laxatives

Adding gentle, stimulating herbs to the diet will correct mild cases of constipation. Purgative herbs possess great value when not overused. Cascara sagrada and rhubarb root are strong laxative herbs that stimulate the secretion of bile flow into the intestines. Demulcent and soothing herbs like licorice and slippery elm bark offer lubrication and mild stimulation of the colon peristalsis.

Gentle Stimulating Tea Formula

> ½ part ginger
> 3 parts licorice
> 2 parts fennel
> 1/8 part senna
> 2 parts slippery elm bark
> 2 parts psyllium seed

Steep 1 teaspoon per cup for 20 minutes and drink three cups per day, or as often as needed. If this stimulating formula does not suffice, add laxative herbs such as cascara sagrada or more senna. Be sure to drink sufficient amounts of water per day.

Cascara sagrada, rhamnus purshiana and cassia senna are common herbs used for constipation. I do not recommend using these herbs over a long period of time or in excessive amounts, especially cascara sagrada, which is very strong. These herbs may be purchased in several forms, including loose herb, fluid extract, capsule and tea.

Psyllium Husks: Plantago ovata or psyllium husks are commonly used for constipation. Psyllium husks are a mucilaginous bulk laxative. A typical dose is one to two teaspoons in a full glass of water, taken twenty minutes before a meal.

Another Flaxseed Suggestion: Flaxseeds are considered to be a bulk, mucilaginous type of laxative, thereby benefiting the condition of constipation. They are high in vitamin F and assist in the healing process. Combine one tablespoon of whole seed to an eight ounce glass of water and let stand until the seeds plump up. In a case study of healthy young adults consuming 50 g flaxseed a day for 4 weeks, bowel movements increased 30 percent per week while flaxseed was consumed.[12]

---

12 Am J Clin Nutr 61 (1), 62-68, 1995.

Exercise

Exercise is an excellent way to reduce stress and help control symptoms of digestive disorders. Many are surprised to learn how exercise can help improve bowel tone. Exercise is an essential element in maintaining a healthy lifestyle. Regular exercise has many benefits, including reduction of fatigue by improving physical stamina, enhancing flexibility, supporting our musculoskeletal system, and reduction of triglyceride and cholesterol levels. Even unwanted habits are lessened through exercise. Exercise improves all aspects of life, including our self image, attitude and appearance.

It is important to find an exercise program that is right for you. There is little risk for most people if they start out with a less vigorous exercise program and increase gradually. Depending upon your age and medical history, a stress test and an electrocardiogram may be advised. In most cases, your body will guard you against potential problems when over-exercising.

For toning and strengthening simultaneously, try exercises like yoga, Tai chi, calisthenics, and weight training. A routine of morning stretching for approximately 20 minutes is a great wake up call. It is a wonderful way to start the day. Aerobic exercise is also beneficial for increasing your heart rate and expanding your lungs. Other choices may include jogging, brisk walking, swimming, climbing stairs, and bicycling. Swimming is probably the most ideal, providing overall fitness while enhancing muscle tone without placing excessive strain on the joints.

The key is movement. Surprisingly, walking a mile will burn as many calories (approximately 100) as jogging a mile. Depending on the weather, consider combining different types of exercise. For instance, indoor stationary exercise bikes, dance classes, yoga or jazzercise classes when the weather is bad. Other recreational exercises might be tennis, golf, hiking, or racquetball. As an added bonus, all of these activities provide an opportunity for meeting new people while obtaining support and encouragement.

When exercising, remember to warm up and cool down after each sequence. Do not be overzealous when beginning an exercise program, apply restraint and sensibility. Build up gradually to more advanced levels.

> TIP: A warm bath with one or two cups of salt (any salt will work) will relax your nervous system and ease muscle pain after exercising. This protocol also works well for insomnia. To increase effect, more salt may be added if desired. This is also a therapy for weaker kidneys to strengthen them in aiding their ability to better absorb minerals.

CHAPTER THIRTEEN

Best Choices for Gluten-Free Grains, Fiber and Foods

Gluten-Free Grains and Products

Maintaining variety in one's diet is one of the many challenges when adopting a gluten-free lifestyle or a gluten-free diet. Begin by acquainting yourself with quality foods and ingredients that do not contain gluten. Nutritional deficiencies can also be a concern; since whole grains are high in B vitamins, minerals, vitamin E, protein and other benefits, removing these from your diet without compensating for the nutritional loss can have ill effects. The dilemma in the past was that most gluten-free products were not whole grain sources; in fact, many remain the same.

Fortunately, the choices available for people living on gluten restricted diets today are vastly different. And the list is growing to include nutritious flours and starches made from grains, rice, beans, nuts and seeds. Whether a person is celiac or gluten intolerant, whole grains should be included in their diet. The following list of examples includes a variety of choices to make one's cooking experience more enjoyable while remaining nutritionally sound.

The gluten-free standard requires that food labeled *gluten-free* contain less than 20 parts per million of gluten. Refer to Chapter 12: "Gluten Alert: FDA Implements New Standards" for detailed information on the new government regulations.

Wild Rice: The labeling of wild rice is similar to that of quinoa. Wild rice is not a grain, but is rather a seed (although botanically, it's closely related to ordinary white rice). As with all other rice, there is no gluten.

Note: There is a rare benefit that wild rice offers to Type 'A' Crohn's patients who cannot eat carbohydrates, but who *can* use wild rice. It is now being introduced in flour form.

Amaranth: In addition to amaranth being safe and gluten-free, its entire plant family has never possessed any gluten in any other member of its species.

Buckwheat: Throughout the U.K. and European countries, buckwheat is used as a gluten-free alternative. Exercise caution when purchasing this flour, as it may contain wheat flour.

Corn (Whole Grain) or Cornmeal: If your body can tolerate it, this grain is very useful, as well as being high in nutrition and gluten-free. Be aware that corn often times triggers an allergic reaction. Care must be taken when considering it for consumption, as mycotoxin, which is associated with corn, is hazardous for those with intestinal disorders.

Millet and Sorghum: Millet and Sorghum are botanically cereal grains, but have been shown to be more closely linked to corn than to sorghum, (whole grain) wheat or rye. As of yet, conclusive tests have not been performed to ensure that these grains are in fact gluten-free. Nevertheless, millet and sorghum are being used in recipes requiring no gluten, and it has been suggested that they do not contain gluten.

Ragi: Also known as Finger millet, African millet and Red millet, ragi is native to Africa and Asia. Ragi may be used by boiling the seeds and can be purchased as flour. When opting for flour, it is best to buy organic to ensure the product's purity. This family of millet is widely used in recipes and favored by gluten restricted persons. Ragi is also considered a staple starch, especially when eaten with its hull, thereby retaining the majority of nutrients such as iron, calcium, antioxidants and a reasonable level of protein. The glycemic index of ragi is high (above 70).

Quinoa: Quinoa is earning a reputation as a very nutritious grain (though it is not actually a grain) and as a great source of protein. Quinoa is 60 percent protein and very versatile to cook with, with applications for breakfast to dinner and even dessert. For this reason, quinoa is a very sought-after alternative to wheat, rye, barley and commercial oats in the diet of gluten sensitive patients, as seen with Crohn's and celiac case. Quinoa's flavor is similar to wild rice, and is slightly nutty. It also contains iron and amino acids such as lysine and sulphuramino acids.

Montina: Milled from Indian rice grass, Montina flour is not a true rice, and its appearance is tan colored with brown flecks. Montina is often used in combination with other gluten-free flours.

Oats: Oats are still dubious for many people with gluten intolerances. To boost your chances, make sure the oats are pure and uncontaminated. Studies are supporting the use of pure, uncontaminated oats in the gluten-free diet—with care.

Rice: Rice is very popular as a grain substitute.

Glutinous Rice: Rice that is categorized as glutinous should not to be confused with the gluten term "glutinous," which means gummy and does not refer to its gluten content. Rice, whether the variety of white rice is described as long grain, short grain, waxy, sweet or glutinous, pertains to the relative amounts of the two types of starch that they contain (amylose and amylopectin).

Rice (Brown, Wild) and Rice Bran are safe and favored among gluten sensitive individuals.

Flax and Hemp Seed: Ground seeds like flax or hemp may be added to other permitted flours or used on their own in baking or cooking. As seeds, they are very nutritious and a good source of protein—a safe and healthy choice to be used freely wherever gluten presents a problem.

Adzuki: Adzuki are small, brown-reddish beans that have a strong nutty taste. They are favored in the macrobiotic diet and with other gluten intolerant diets. Adzuki flour and beans are popular in Japanese cuisine and can be purchased at Asian markets. These beans are commonly used in pastries or with other grains as a main meal.

Teff: Teff is a very small grain, harvested exclusively in Ethiopia for thousands of years, and was virtually unknown to the rest of the world until recently. Teff is gluten-free, highly nutritious and rich in protein, calcium and iron. Teff is now being grown in Idaho, with distribution throughout the country.

Job's Tears: Also referred to as coix seed, the name Job's tears was so given because of its distinctive teardrop shape. Job's tears hail from the grasses in tropical Asia. Like many other Asian cooking products, you may find Job's tears at many oriental markets. It is customarily used like rice or barley (its flavor is closer to that of barley and is gluten-free).

Soy: The legume soy is well known as being gluten-free and comes in several forms for cooking. This is one of the great advantages soy has over many other products, with accessibility being another—it is easy to find. Being a vegetable protein is also a plus, widening its applications even further.

Additional Gluten-Free Flours and Thickeners

> Artichoke flour
>
> Black and red rice (rare Asian rice)
>
> Beans and seeds of leguminous plants (flour and thickeners)
>
> Chickpea flour, dal (chickpeas)
>
> Cassava root flour (tapioca, manioc, yucca)
>
> Calrose rice
>
> Carolina gold rice
>
> Cottonseed flour
>
> Coffee flour
>
> Chestnut roasted (flour)
>
> Dasheen flour (taro)

Della rice

Jasmine rice (aromatic)

Maize, masa, harina (corn)

Milo (flour or cracked)

Peanut flour

Potato flour and starch

Rice (races, called indica, javonica, and sinica (grass family))

Rice bran (outer layer of brown rice)

Sago starch (extracted from tropical palms)

Sweet potato (dried and ground into flour)

Taro flour (thickener, similar to tapioca)

Texmati rice (aromatic)

Valencia rice

Water chestnut (dried and ground into a flour)

Wehani rice (California hybrid rice)

Wild pecan rice (aromatic from Louisiana)

Gluten-Free Plant Fiber

Dietary plant fiber offers many health benefits and is a replacement for the glutinous properties provided by gluten:

Crude fiber is composed of a starch-like molecule called cellulose, a polysaccharide, which is a carbohydrate polymer of D-glucose. Cellulose is the non-digestible plant structure found in the skin of fruits and vegetables and other material in plants. Cellulose does not contain gluten protein.

Sources of crude fiber include all legumes, cereals, fruit, and vegetables (in particular, root vegetables and cabbage), all plants in general, and the hulls of seeds and the skin on apples.

Hemicelluloses are known for the gum property found in the cell walls of plants. This carbohydrate is related to cellulose, which is also a polysaccharide, whose primary importance is its ability to absorb water.

Hemicellulose is present in cereals, bran, whole grains and the legume family.

Pectin is a type of *hemicellulose* used in commercial jellies and jams. Pectin can be found in apples, strawberries, and citrus fruits.

Methyl cellulose is a chemically converted composition of cellulose, and is therefore not a naturally occurring molecule found in the plant itself. This form of cellulose has great applications as a good substitute for gluten in rice-based breads and other gluten-free substances. Psyllium fiber is similar in nature to methylcellulose; both are derived from natural sources. The husks and seeds are used from the plant *Plantago ovata* (or blond psyllium) to produce psyllium fiber. These fibers, like others, become gelatinous when mixed with water.

Lignin is not considered to be a carbohydrate, even though it is of plant origin. Also known as crude fiber, lignin is the principal element in the woody structure of plants. Lignin is a primary component of the secondary cell walls in plants and some algae. Lignin occupies the space in the cell wall between hemicellulose, cellulose, and pectin.

Sources in food will vary; however, examples include the seeds of fruits, root vegetables and vegetables with filaments such as celery and string beans, and also cereals.

Lignans are classified as a group of *phytoestrogens* (not to be confused with lignin). Lignans are one of the major sources of plant estrogens (phytoestrogen) and act as antioxidants. These estrogen-type compounds are metabolized by intestinal bacteria of mammalian lignans, enterodiol and enterolactone. Other categories of phytoestrogens are isoflavones and courmestans. Plant lignans are a constituent of dietary fiber.

Sources from food include flax seeds and sesame seeds, which each contain higher amounts of lignans than most other foods. Look to nuts and seeds like pumpkin, sunflower, poppy, cashew and peanuts to boost your lignans intake. Other rich sources include grains like rye, oats and wheat, as well as soybeans and soy products. Vegetables richer in lignans are found in the cruciferous family, such as cabbage (red and white), broccoli, kale, cauliflower and Brussels sprouts, as well as carrots and green and red peppers. Fruits and vegetables are typically lower in lignans as compared to other sources, but of those, strawberries and apricots are particularly good sources, with others including peaches, pears, pink grapefruit, cherries and nectarines.

Chitosan is related to a group of carbohydrates called amino polysaccharides. Today, chitosan is used for its many health benefiting characteristics, including as a well-researched source of soluble dietary fiber. This fiber product is derived from the shells of shrimp, crabs, oyster shells and the cell walls of fungi, and has demonstrated great benefits for lowering cholesterol.

Glucomannan or **konjac mannan** is another important dietary carbohydrate fiber substance. Konjac root powder or flour is used for controlling diabetic sugar levels because of its ability to prevent the rapid uptake of glucose in the small intestine. Guar gum is also part of the mannan family. Other areas of use are in aiding weight loss and lowering cholesterol levels.

Vegetable gum fiber, such as guar gum and acacia Senegal gum are often sold in loose powder form or in a capsule. Other fibers that would be closely related as (far as consistency) are locust bean and pectin. These are very gentle, forming a jelly-like texture with no aftertaste.

Plants Related to Wheat that May be Tolerated by Celiac Patients

Recent patient testimonials and clinical trials have suggested that foods which are very distantly related to wheat may not pose a problem for celiac patients. For instance, buckwheat, quinoa, amaranth, and rapeseed oil (canola) fall into this category. Still, it may be possible for some celiac and other patients with gut disorders to have an allergic or other adverse reaction to these grains, or foodstuffs containing such items. Be that as it may, there is currently no scientific basis for saying that these allergies, or other adverse reactions, have anything to do with gluten intolerance. An example would be if a patient who is lactose intolerant or has an allergy to milk proteins, doesn't necessarily have an adverse reaction to milk.

Grain Samples to Avoid

Spelt (or Spelta) and Kamut fall within the wheat family. They contain gluten, which is toxic to celiac patients and should be avoided. Other examples include breads using wheat, durum wheat, rye, barley, and triticale.

Caution: Recently, there have been claims that the cereal grain spelt can be used as an ingredient in the diets of those who suffer with celiac disease and other such aliments. Note that the basis for this claim has not been substantiated.

Bulgur (Burghul): Bulgur is wheat that has gone through a process of being parboiled, then dried and cracked. This grain must be avoided by persons with gluten intolerance.

Semolina: Semolina is derived from wheat and is considered a highly gluten product. Semolina must be avoided.

Other Related Items from Wheat Sources

Dinkle

Faro

Couscous

Durum

Einkorn

Farina

Fu (Wheat)

Freekeh (Middle Eastern wheat cereal)

Gliadin (gluten peptide)

Graham

Khorasan (ancient variety of wheat)

Matza

Mir (wheat and rye)

Seitan (wheat gluten)

Triticale

Note: Rice bran, wild rice and corn (maize) are not toxic to celiac patients.

Gluten-Free Flours

Popular Flour List
These diverse flour choices are compiled in order of popular choice, by supply and demand of product retailers.

1. Almond flour
2. Organic coconut flour (gluten-free)
3. Gluten-free sweet white sorghum flour
4. Tapioca flour
5. Organic rice flour (brown)
6. Natural almond flour
7. Chestnut flour
8. Chickpea flour
9. Millet flour
10. Chia flour
11. Organic quinoa flour
12. Organic amaranth flour
13. Hazelnut flour
14. Gluten-free sweet white rice flour
15. Peanut flour
16. Pumpkin seed powder
17. Teff flour
18. Organic almond flour
19. Pistachio flour
20. Cashew flour
21. White chia flour
22. Organic rice flour (white)
23. Gluten-free garbanzo fava flour
24. Potato flour
25. Gluten-free masa harina corn flour
26. Sprouted super flour
27. Gluten-free corn flour
28. Gluten-free green pea flour
29. Gluten-free white bean flour
30. Gluten-free black bean flour
31. Gluten-free fava bean flour

Get free celiac.com email alerts (1–3 emails per month) with the latest celiac disease research and information and gluten-free recipes.

List of Gluten-Free Ingredients and Foods

Safe Gluten-Free Food List (Safe Ingredients)
Reprinted by permission of www.celiac.com

Acorn quercus
Adzuki bean
Agar
Agave
Alcohol (specific
    spirits types)
Alfalfa
Algae
Almond nut
Amaranth
Ambergris
Apple cider vinegar
Arrowroot
Artichokes
Artificial butter flavor
Aspic
Autolyzed yeast extract
Avena sativia (oats 3)
Avena sativia extract
Baking soda
Balsamic vinegar
Beans
Bean, adzuki
Bean, hyacinth
Bean, lentil
Bean, mung
Bean romano
    (chickpea)

Bean tepary
Besan (chickpea)
Bicarbonate of soda
Blue cheese
Brown sugar
Buckwheat
Butter (check
    additives)
Cane sugar
Cane vinegar
Canola (rapeseed)
Canola oil (rapeseed)
Carbonated water
Carob bean
Carob bean gum
Carob flour
Carrageenan
Casein
Cassava
Champagne vinegar
Channa (chickpea)
Chana flour (chickpea)
Cheeses (most, but
    check ingredients)
Chestnuts
Chickpea
Chlorella
Chocolate liquor

Cochineal
Cocoa
Cocoa butter
Coconut
Confectioner's glaze
Corn
Corn gluten
Corn masa flour
Corn meal
Corn flour
Corn starch
Corn sugar
Corn syrup
Corn sweetener
Corn vinegar
Cotton seed
Cotton seed oil
Cowitch
Cowpea
Cream of tartar
Crospovidone
Curds
Dal (lentils)
Dasheen flour (taro)
Dates
Delactosed whey
Distilled alcohols
Dutch processed cocoa

Eggs
Fish (fresh)
Flaked rice
Flax
Fruit (including dried)
Fruit vinegar
Garbanzo beans
Gelatin
Glutinous rice
Glutinous rice flour
Gram flour (chick
   peas)
Grape skin extract
Grits, corn
Hemp
Hemp seeds
Herbs
Herb vinegar
Hominy
Honey
Hops
Horseradish (pure)
Hyacinth bean
Meat protein
Isolated soy protein
Job's tears
Jowar (sorghum)
Kasha
Koshihikari (rice)
Kudzu
Kudzu root starch
Lard
Lemon grass
Lentils
Licorice
Licorice extract
Locust bean gum
Maize

Masa flour
Masa harina
Meat (fresh)
Milk
Milk protein isolate
Millet
Milo (sorghum)
Msg
Mung bean
Mustard flour
Non-fat milk
Nuts
Oils and fats
Paprika
Peas
Pea (chickpeas)
Pea (cowpeas)
Pea flour
Pea starch
Peanuts
Peanut flour
Pectin
Peppers
Pigeon peas
Polenta
Potatoes
Potato flour
Potato starch
Povidone
Prinus
Propolis
Psyllium
Quinoa
Ragi
Rape
Rice
Rice (enriched)
Rice flour

Rice starch
Rice syrup
Rice vinegar
Romano bean
   (chickpea)
Saffron
Sago
Sago palm
Sago flour
Sago starch
Saifun (bean threads)
Salt
Seaweed
Seeds
Seed (sesame)
Seed (sunflower)
Soba (be sure it is 100
   percent buckwheat)
Sorghum
Sorghum flour
Soy
Soybean
Soy lecithin
Soy protein
Soy protein isolate
Spices (pure)
Spirits (specific types)
Stevia
Sunflower seed
Succotash (corn and
   beans)
Sucrose
Sweet chestnut flour
Tallow
Tapioca
Tapioca flour
Tapioca starch
Taro

Tarro

Tarrow root

Tea

Tea-tree oil

Teff

Teff flour

Tepary bean

Textured vegetable
    protein

Tofu (soy curd)

Torula yeast

Turmeric

Urad/urid beans

Urad/urid dal (peas)

Urad/urid flour

Urd

Vinegar (all except
    malt)

Vanilla extract

Vanilla flavoring

Vanillin

Whey

Whey protein
    concentrate

Whey protein isolate

Wines

Wild rice

Yam flour

Yeast

Yogurt (plain,
    unflavored)

CHAPTER FOURTEEN

Conclusion

WE ARE LIVING in an age where patients are no longer satisfied with being patted on the head, patronized, and sent away from their physician's office with unanswered questions. In health care today, patients are frequently and rightfully demanding to know the details of tests being performed, why they are necessary and what other options may be available. Decisions and treatment should *involve* the patient, enabling them to participate and have a full understanding of their diagnosis and any subsequent procedures.

Modern civilization has adversely affected the health of our bowels, as well as many other aspects of our health and well-being. A large part of the population is not concerned with quality of life, or making healthier food choices. Add to that, unhealthy lifestyles and living habits are resulting in bodies that cannot eliminate properly, and which invite common and oftentimes chronic health circumstances, as seen in constipation and diverticulosis. Our body is only as clean as our bowels; proper assimilation of vital nutrients cannot take place through build-up of the bowel wall. The bowel becomes overwhelmed by toxin-producing bacteria and viruses, which eventually accumulate in inherently weak areas of the body.

There is no single conclusive test available to diagnose gastrointestinal disorders. Laboratory diagnostic studies, such as a sigmoidoscopy, leaky gut test, blood tests and stool specimen, etc., are performed to help determine the patient's type of disorder. There are a host of symptoms and complications accompanying bowel complaints that are also taken into consideration.

For example, Crohn's disease and ulcerative colitis are similar in symptoms, with a major difference: Crohn's disease, or regional enteritis, may affect *any* segment of the digestive tract, from the esophagus to the anus.

Ulcerative colitis and other forms of colitis are limited to the colon and rectum. Celiac patients react primarily to gluten, and sometimes dairy products. Irritable bowel syndrome is the most common of all the digestive disorders and has many names—spastic colitis, nervous stomach, spastic colon, mucous colitis, among others. Constipation is not considered a disease, although it marks the start of many problems (such as diverticulitis). An impacted colon may also lead to more serious problems such as cancer.

Extensive research and countless testimonials of individuals suffering from digestive disorders show a direct correlation between diet and gastrointestinal problems. Alternative treatments address autoimmune disorders or food allergies through diet, nutritional supplementation, herbal medicine, and lifestyle changes.

One example of addressing these sorts of complications *without* resorting to medication is by taking better command of the carbohydrates in our diet. Carbohydrates (referring to starch and disaccharide sugar molecules) require digestion before absorption. Undigested carbohydrates ferment within the intestine, influencing microbial overgrowth. Harmful intestinal bacteria injure the intestinal wall, destroying enzymes, while increasing the production of gas, acids, yeasts and mucus (all of which enhance malabsorption). By incorporating certain carbohydrates which require minimal digestion, we stop feeding the harmful bacteria in our gut and thus improve nourishment. Once this destructive cycle begins to reverse, the body no longer needs protection from noxious bacteria. Mucous production is then reduced and carbohydrate digestion improves, replacing malabsorption with absorption.

Emotional stress is another player, serving as both a main and a contributing factor to intestinal disorders. Added to this are physical factors, such as food sensitivities, which must be investigated to fully determine the causes of all gut dysbiosis. Two of the most common food intolerances are lactose (milk sugar) and gluten (the protein in grains). Inflammatory bowel disease research has produced remarkable results related to the removal of carbohydrates in the diet. These studies involve the elimination of foods and beverages containing carbohydrates, especially food items in the form of starches and sucrose. Other studies yielded the same dramatic results and sustained remissions using an elimination diet of specific substances, mainly found in the food groups of cereals and dairy products.

Cleansing and eliminating regimens are highly beneficial in maintaining good health and conquering physical illness. Malnourishment is common among people suffering from inflammatory bowel disease. Supplementation is necessary to combat nutrient loss through an insufficient diet, malabsorption, diarrhea, pain and nausea.

Dietary influences also play a paramount role in intestinal disorders. More awareness and education is needed, both among physicians and in the general public. Most gastroenterologists, despite the research findings, *still* do not consider the diet of individuals they are treating. A small but growing percentage of the public are gradually becoming aware of the importance of diet in preventive health care. We cannot buy good health; we must earn it, or rather *learn* it.

The standard Western diet is high in fat, high in carbohydrates, and rich in highly processed foods with many additives and preservatives. It is also the root cause of many digestive disorders (coupled with nutrient deficiencies). It amazes me that people feel they can call upon their bodies to perform when their level of nourishment is so substandard. The general public is blindly unaware as to what our bodies require to rebuild and function at an optimum level. This is not the fault of the general public; *none* of us can make quality decisions about what is required to keep us well if appropriate information is never provided to us at a time when it would serve us best. During our traditional academic years, when we are a captive audience and most receptive to this vital information, is when we should be taught how to provide our bodies with what they desperately need.

Our digestive system is as individualized as we are, and needs to be treated on an individual basis. The information on diet today offers new hope for all people who suffer from intestinal disorders. To achieve and sustain normalcy is attainable for many, through proper management of diet and lifestyle.

SAMPLE

CROHN'S DISEASE AND GASTROINTESTINAL COMPLAINT QUESTIONNAIRE

NAME: _____

ADDRESS: _____

PHONE: HOME: _____WORK: _____

EMAIL: _____

AGE: _____   ____MALE: ____FEMALE:

OCCUPATIONS: _____

PROVIDE ANY AVAILABLE BLOOD WORK OR OTHER MEDICAL TESTS:

_____

_____

_____

LIST OF HEALTH COMPLAINTS (LIST FROM MAJOR TO MINOR):

_____

_____

_____

_____

_____

About Hyperbaric Oxygen Treatment (HBOT)

* Hyperbaric Oxygen Treatment (HBOT): Under normal conditions, 97.5 percent of oxygen is carried in the bloodstream bound to hemoglobin and the remaining 2.5 percent is dissolved in plasma. Traditional uses: decompression sickness, air embolism, carbon monoxide poisoning, acute traumatic ischemia (crush injuries that deprive tissues of oxygen), and bacterial invasion of a necrotic wound (tissue has died). HBOT is a technique of delivering 100 percent oxygen directly to an open, moist wound.

* The topical HBOT oxygen device consists of an appliance to enclose the wound area (frequently an extremity) and a source of oxygen. Conventional oxygen tanks may be used.

* Topical HBOT has been explored as a treatment of skin ulcerations due to diabetes, venous stasis, post-surgical infection, gangrenous lesion, decubitus ulcers, amputation, skin graft, burns or frostbite.

1. How long have you had these symptoms?

2. How many oxygen treatments, if any?

3. What degree of success?

4. Did your mother have measles during her pregnancy with you?

5. Have you had surgery?

6. Where is your inflammation located?

7. What supplements are you taking?

8. Do you have a sweet tooth?

9. How severe is your gas, bloating, diarrhea or abdominal pain?

10. What foods cause gas, bloating, diarrhea, or abdominal pain?

11. How many servings of starches and sugars do you eat in a day? List them?

12. How many vegetables? List them?

13. How many fruits? List them?

14. How many proteins? List them?

15. How many dairy products? List them?

16. How many drinks? List them?

17. How much junk food? List them?

18. Did you have recurrent antibiotic pneumonia preceded by Crohn's symptoms in every case? *(Note: Antibiotics are known to increase fungal infection. Most antibiotics are mycotoxins-fungal derivatives. Mycotoxins are found in our grain food. Anyone who has consumed antibiotics, grains or sugars has a comprised immune system.)*

19. Have you gone through severe emotional stress?

20. Did your symptoms exist before the stress?

21. Do you have leaky gut?

22. Do you have any allergies? Name them.

23. Do you smoke?

Please list any and all medication you are currently taking, or have recently taken: _____

_____

_____

_____

_____

_____

_____

_____

CELIAC DISEASE CRITICAL RESEARCH AREAS

- CFCR Discovers the Difference between CD and Gluten Sensitivity (GS): Research provides the first evidence of a different mechanism leading to GS. The study also demonstrates that GS and CD are part of a spectrum of gluten-related disorders.
- Gluten Spectrum Disorders Identified: Dr. Fasano chairs a committee to define the difference between a wheat allergy, gluten sensitivity and CD.
- Update on Zonulin: Dr. Fasano's article, "Zonulin and Its Regulation of Intestinal Barrier Function: The Biological Door to Inflammation, Autoimmunity, and Cancer," presents a detailed account of the intriguing role that zonulin plays in the development of a host of diseases.
- Innate Immune Study and Chemotaxis Study: The CFCR is currently investigating the body's natural response to gliadin in people with CD and gluten sensitivity to identify the very early event(s) responsible for the development of gluten spectrum disorders. Understanding these pathways may offer new preventive and therapeutic strategies for CD and possibly other autoimmune diseases.
- Infant Nutrition and Risk of Celiac Disease: Work continues on this study and has enrolled over 750 babies worldwide to examine whether delaying the introduction of gluten to an infant's diet may prevent the onset of CD in genetically at-risk infants. If you are interested in this study, please email glutenproject@peds.umaryland.edu.
- Possible Link between Schizophrenia and CD/GS: The CFCR continues to investigate this link, and preliminary observations suggest that 1 out of 5 could be affected by gluten sensitivity and, therefore, can potentially benefit from a gluten-free diet.
- Microbiome and Risk of Gluten-Related Disorders: The Chemotaxis and Autism Speaks Studies are looking at the changes in the normal internal flora and how that may relate to the development of celiac disease, gluten sensitivity and autism.

- Possible Link Between Autism and CD/GS: The CFCR is investigating a link between autism and gluten sensitivity. This study could potentially help identify the individuals with autism and gluten sensitivity that might benefit from a gluten-free diet.
- Celiac Disease Research Registry: The CFCR's celiac disease registry continues to expand, which will enable us to learn more about gluten-related disorders, their complications and co-morbidities.
- Update on Alba Therapeutics: The CFCR continues to focus some of its research activities to develop alternative/integrated strategies to the gluten-free diet. Our efforts continue to provide the rationale for Alba Therapeutics to perform the clinical trials necessary to exploit these strategies.

HERBAL REMEDIES:
ADDITIONAL RESEARCH RESOURCES

54 Herb Society Forum
www.network54.com

Herbs are Special
http://www.herbsarespecial.com.au/free-herb-information/comfrey.html#

Herb Craft
www.theherbcraft.org/hoffmann.comfrey.html

Natural Standards Database
http://3rdparty.naturalstandard.com/frameset.asp

Cochrane Database Systems Reviews
http://community.cochrane.org/editorial-and-publishing-policy-resource/
cochrane-database-systematic-reviews-cdsr

National Institutes of Health
https://nccih.nih.gov/

The National Institutes of Health (NIH) is a biomedical research facility primarily located in Bethesda, Maryland. An agency of the United States Department of Health and Human Services, it is the primary agency of the United States government responsible for biomedical and health-related research. The NIH both conducts its own scientific research through its Intramural Research Program (IRP) and provides major biomedical research funding to non-NIH research facilities through its Extramural Research Program.

National Center for Complementary and Alternative Medicine
https://nccih.nih.gov/

Herbs-at-a-Glance
https://nccih.nih.gov/health/herbsataglance.htm

Ayurvedic Medicine
https://nccih.nih.gov/health/ayurveda/introduction.htm

American Botanical Council ABC
http://abc.herbalgram.org/site/PageServer

Natural Database Therapeutic Research
http://naturaldatabase.therapeuticresearch.com/home.aspx?cs=&s=ND

National Institutes of Health Office of Dietary Supplements
http://ods.od.nih.gov/

American Herbalists Guild
http://www.americanherbalistsguild.com/

The College of Practitioners of Phytotherapy
http://www.phytotherapists.org/

Herb Research Foundation
http://www.herbs.org/herbnews/

International Herb Association
http://www.iherb.org/

National Institute of Medical Herbalists
http://www.nimh.org.uk/

BIBLIOGRAPHY

Introduction

Celiac Reference: Fasano et al. (2003)

Crohn's and Ulcerative Colitis: Reference: Can. J. Gastroneterol Nov. 2010; 24(11): 651-655.

Wolever, Thomas MS, Peter J. Spadafora 1995; American Journal of Clinical Nutrition; Propionate inhibits incorporation of colonic acetate, vol. 61; 1241-1247

Chapter 1

Airola, Paavo 1990; How To Get Well; Constipation, 64; Colitis, 62; Diverticulosis, 80; Health Plus, Publishers, Sherwood, Oregon

Phillips, Jode, Jane G. Muir 1995; American Journal of Clinical Nutrition; Resistant starch on fecal bulk and fermentation, vol. 62:121-130

Robbins, John 1987; Diet For A New America; Constipation, 284-287; Diverticulosis, 285-287; Irritable Bowel Syndrome, 286-287; Stillpoint Publishing, Walpole, NH 03608

Roberfroid, Bornet F. 1996; International Clinical Nutrition Review; Colonic microflora, vol. 16: (January), 154-155

Clinical Dietitian, SickKids Hospital -Canada's Food Guide has specific recommendations about the amount of grain we should be eating each day. It also recommends that 50 percent of the grains we consume should be whole grains.

Dr. J.A. Campbell; Acceptability of Grains and Other - Foods Canadian Celiac Association. Dr. J. A. Campbell (1923–1993) worked in the Federal Department of Agriculture, the Drug Directorate of the Department of National Health and Welfare, and became Director of the Nutrition Bureau, Health Protection Branch in 1972, where he was officer-in-charge of the Nutrition Canada Survey.

Fasano A, Berti I, Gerarduzzi T, Not T, Colletti R, Drago S, Elitsur Y, Green P, Guandalini S, Hill I, Pietzak M, Ventura A, Thorpe M, Kryszak D, Fornaroli F, Wasserman S, Murray J, Horvath K (2003). "Prevalence of celiac disease in at-risk and not-at-risk groups in the United States: a large multicenter study." Archives of Internal Medicine 163 (3): 286–92. doi:10.1001/archinte.163.3.286. PMID 12578508.

Haas SV (1924). "The value of the banana in the treatment of coeliac disease." Am J Dis Child 24: 421–37.

"Increased Prevalence and Mortality in Undiagnosed Celiac Disease." Gastroenterology 137 (1): 88–93. doi:10.1053/j.gastro.2009.03.059. PMC 2704247. PMID 19362553.

Stephen, Alison M., Wendy J. Glynis 1995; American Journal of Clinical Nutrition; Colonic function, vol. 62; 1261-1267

Varela-Moreiras G, Murphy MM, Scott JM (May 2009). "Cobalamin, folic acid, and homocysteine." Nutrition Reviews 67 (Suppl 1): S69–72. doi:10.1111/j.1753-4887.2009.00163.x. PMID 19453682.

Chapter 2

Mills, Simon Steven J. Finando 1989; Alternatives In Healing; Digestive and Endocrine systems, 106-107; New American Library, New York and Scarborough Ontario

Dunne, Lavon 1990; Nutrition Almanac Third Edition; McGraw-Hill, Publishing Company

Balas, E A. (2001). "Information Systems Can Prevent Errors and Improve Quality." Journal of the American Medical Informatics Association 8 (4): 398–9. doi:10.1136/jamia.2001.0080398. PMC 130085. PMID 11418547.

Bindra A, Braunstein GB. Thyroiditis. Am Fam Physician. 2006;73(10):1769-76.

Duntas LH. Environmental factors and autoimmune thyroiditis. Nat Clin Pract Endocrinol Metab. 2008;4(8)454-60.

"Diagnosis of hypothyroidism: Are we getting what we want from TSH testing?" The Non-Profit National Academy of Hypothyroidism. Nahypothyroidism.org. Retrieved 2014-06-29.

"How Accurate is TSH Testing?" NAHypothyroidism.org. Retrieved 2014-06-29.

"Why Doesn't My Endocrinologist Know All Of This?" The Non-Profit National Academy of Hypothyroidism. Nahypothyroidism.org. Retrieved 2014-07-12. (This article was also part-published in "The Pituitary Network.")

Chapter 3

Browning, James E. 1996; Journal of the Neuromusculoskeletal System; (PROD) Pelvic pain and organic dysfunction, vol. 4; #2, 52-56.

Reference: Prevalence of Diverticular Disease: 2 million people in the USA 1983-87 (Digestive diseases in the United States: Epidemiology and Impact–NIH Publication No. 94-1447, NIDDK, 1994) ... see also overview of Diverticular Disease. Incidence (annual) of Diverticular Disease: 300,000 new cases in the USA 1987 (Digestive diseases in the United States: Epidemiology and Impact–NIH Publication No. 94-1447, NIDDK, 1994)

References: The American Journal of Gastroenterology, ISSN: 0002-9270, EISSN: 1572-0241; © 2014 The American College of Gastroenterology.*The Prevalence of Celiac Disease in the United States: Alberto Rubio-Tapia, Jonas F Ludvigsson, Tricia L Brantner, Joseph A Murray and James E Everhart.

Chopra, Deepak 1994; Alternative Medicine; Gastrointestinal Disorders, 680-689; Constipation, 640-645; Future Medicine Publishing Inc., Puyallup WA. 98371

Cummings, John H., Hans N. Englyst 1995; American Journal of Clinical Nutrition; Gastrointestinal effects of food carbohydrate; vol. 61; 938S-945S

Donovan, Patrick 1996; Textbook Of Natural Medicine; Bowel Toxaemia, Permeability and Disease, IV: BwTox-1-7; Bastyr University Publishing, Bothell, Washington

Jensen, Bernard 1983; Food Healing For Man; Colitis, 18-, 130, 198, 316, 364; Constipation, 35, 169-170, 300-301, 357; Diverticulosis, 169-171, 353-354; Bernard Jensen Enterprises, Escondido, CA

Fasano A (2009). "Celiac Disease Insights: Clues to Solving Autoimmunity." Scientific American (August): 49–57.

Chapter 4

Mukherjee, Debasis 1994; The Homeopathic Heritage; Bowel Nosodes, vol. 19: 409-411

Murray, Michael T., Joseph E. Pizzorno; Encyclopedia Of Natural Medicine; Constipation, 232-254; Crohn's Disease and Ulcerative colitis, 237-254; Irritable Bowel Syndrome, 395-400; Prima Publishing, Rocklin, CA. 95677

Galland, L. Leaky Gut Syndromes: Breaking the Vicious Cycles. Townsend Letter for Doctors 145:62 (1995, Aug/Sept). Toxins of many kinds can increase intestinal permeability. These include alcohol, nonsteroidal anti-inflammatory drugs (aspirin, ibuprofen, arthritis medications, and many others), cytotoxic drugs used to treat cancer, corticosteroid drugs, and, by their action on bowel flora, antibiotics.

Chapter 5

J. Anderson and S. Perryman, "Dietary Fiber," Colorado State University Extension, May 2007, http://ext.colostate.edu/pubs/foodnut/09333html

Carrie, H. S. Ruxton, Elaine J. Gardner and Drew Walker, "Can Pure Fruit and Vegetable Juices Protect Against Cancer and Cardiovascular Disease Too?" Internal Journal of Food Sciences and Nutrition 57 (May 2006): 249-272.

Jeanie Lerche Davis, "Fruits and Veggies Lower Blood Pressure," WebMD. com, May 28, 2002, http://www.webmd.com/diet/news/2002528/fruits-veggies-lower-blood-pressure

Anthony Wilson, "Carotenoids in Fruits and Vegetables May Cut Arthritis Risk," Arthritis News, Articles and Information, March 12, 2008.http://www.healthhubs.net/arthritis/carotenoids-in-fruits-vegetables-may-cut-arthritis-risk.

Szabo, "Plant foods to the Rescue."

Chapter 6

Kelvinson R.C. 1995; Complementary Therapies In Medicine; Colonic Hydrotherapy, vol. 3: 88-92.

Chapter 7

Garlic, University of Maryland Medical Center (UMMC) Complementary and Alternative Medicine Index (CAM) 2008. http://www.umm.edu/altmed/articles/garlic.000245#Supporting 20 percent Research

J. Voyich et al. Insights into mechanisms used by staphylococcus aureus to avoid destruction by human neutrophils. The Journal of Immunology 175 (6):3907-19 (2005)

Eric Yarnall, Kathy Abascal, Herbal Support for Methicillin-Resistant Staphylococcus aureus Infections. August 2009, Vol. 15.No. 4-189-195

Allen, P, LANCET 2001, 358(9289)1245: Janssen AM et al,. Antimicrobial activity of essential oils. Planta Med 53(5)395-398.

Dr. Keith Courtenay (Metaphysics U.L.C., U.S.A.) Colloidal Silver: The Hidden Truths 2007.

Allen K.L.:Hutchinson, G.:Molan, P.C. The potential for using honey to treat wounds, infected with MRSA and URE (8kb PDF file) 10-13, Sept.2000.

Retrieved Feb. 2. 2012. Published: Nov.25 2008, Telegraph Media Group, UK. Health Alternative Medicine Oregano could help eradicate MRSA superbug.

W4, Tyski S2. Evaluation of biocidal properties of silver nanoparticles against cariogenic bacteria. Med Dosw Mikrobiol. 2013;65(3):197-206.

Coburn Huebner, Y. Ding, I. Petermann, C. Knapp, L. R. Ferguson. The Probiotic Escherichia coli Nissle 1917 Reduces Pathogen Invasion and Modulates Cytokine Expression in Caco-2 Cells Infected with Crohn's Disease-Associated E. coli LF82. Applied and Environmental Microbiology, 2011; 77 (7): 2541 DOI: 10.1128/AEM.01601-10

Nabandith V et al. "Inhibitory effects of crude alpha-mangostin, a xanthone derivative, on two different categories of colon preneoplastic lesions induced by 1, 2-dimethylhydrazine in the rat." Asian Pacific Journal of Cancer Prevention. 5.4 (2004): 433-8.

Sutherlandia: BMC Complementary and Alternative Medicine (Impact Factor: 1.88). 09/2014; 14(1):329. DOI: 10.1186/1472-6882-14-329 Source: PubMed

Gupta, I. (1997). Effects of Boswellia serrata gum resin in patients with ulcerative colitis. Eur J Med Res, 2(1):37-43.

Chapter 8

Thompson L, Spiller RC. 1996; International Clinical Nutrition Review; Colonic Bacterial Metabolism, (January), vol.16, 179-180.

Appleton KM, Hayward RC, Gunnell D, et al. (December 2006). "Effects of n-3 long-chain polyunsaturated fatty acids on depressed mood: systematic review of published trials." Am. J. Clin. Nutr. 84 (6): 1308–16. PMID 17158410.

Akhondzadeh A, Naghavi H, Vazirian M, Shayeganopour A, Rashidi H, Khani M. 2001. Passionflower in the treatment of generalized anxiety: a pilot double blind randomized controlled trial with Oxazepam. J Clin Pharm Ther 26:363-367.

Akhondzadeh, D. Mohammadi, M, Momeni F, 2005. Passiflora incarnata in the treatment of attention deficit hyperactivity disorder in children and adolescents. Therapy 2:609-614.

Akhondzadeh S, Kashani L, Mobaseri M, Hosseini S, Nikzad S, Khani M. 2001 Passionflower in the treatment of opiates withdrawal: a double-blind randomized controlled trial. J Clin Pharm Ther 26:369-373.

Blumenthal M, 1998. The Complete German Commission E Monographs. Therapeutic Guide to Herbal Medicines. Austin: American Botanical Council.

British Herbal Medicine Association. 1996. British Herbal Pharmacopoeia (BHP). Exeter, UK.

Szegedi A, Kohnen R, Dienel A, Kieser M. Acute treatment of moderate to severe depression with hypericum extract WS 5570 (St John's wort): randomized controlled double blind non-inferiority trial versus paroxetine. British Medical Journal 2005 Feb.

Petersen Shay, K, Moreau, RF, Smith, EJ, Hagen, TM (June 2008). "Is alpha-lipoic acid a scavenger of reactive oxygen species in vivo? Evidence for its initiation of stress signaling pathways that promote endogenous antioxidant capacity." IUBMB life 60 (6): 362–7. doi:10.1002/iub.40. PMID 18409172.

Taylor MJ, Wilder H, Bhagwagar Z, Geddes J (2004). Taylor, Matthew J. ed. "Inositol for depressive disorders." Cochrane Database Syst Rev (2): CD004049. doi:10.1002/14651858.CD004049.pub2. PMID 15106232

Thompson MA, Bauer BA, Loehrer LL, et al. (May 2009). "Dietary supplement S-adenosyl-L-methionine (AdoMet) effects on plasma homocysteine levels in healthy human subjects: a double-blind, placebo-controlled, randomized clinical trial." J Altern Complement Med 15 (5): 523–9. doi:10.1089/acm.2008.0402. PMC 2875864. PMID 19422296.

Chen ML, et al. Chemical and biological differentiation of Cortex Phellodendri Chinensis and Cortex Phellodendri Amurensis. Planta Med. (2010)

Kuhn MA, Winston D. Herbal Therapy and Supplements. Philadelphia, Pa: Lippincott; 2001.

Bisset NG. Herbal Drugs and Phytopharmaceuticals. Stuttgart, Germany: Medpharm Scientific Publishers; 2004:534-536.

Source: Willow bark | University of Maryland Medical Center http://umm. edu/health/medical/altmed/herb/willow-bark#ixzz3OkX5UcW8

Singh N, Hoette Y. Tulsi: the mother medicine of nature. Lucknow, India: International Institute of Herbal Medicine, 2002.

Arteaga A, Santa-Olalla P, Sierra MJ, Limia A, Cortes M, Amela C. [Epidemic risk of disease associated with a new strain of Clostridium difficile.] Enfermedades Infecciosas y Microbiologia Clinica Epub ahead of print (2009). Clostridium difficile (C. dificile) infections have increased in North America and Europe over the last few decades, mostly as a result of antibiotic abuse. A new strain of C. difficile, known as toxigenic type III, has increased pathogenicity and antibiotic resistance resulting in the threat of an epidemic if immediate steps are not taken. PubMed Reference PMID:19386385

Turner EH, Blackwell AD (2005). "5-Hydroxytryptophan plus SSRIs for interferon-induced depression: synergistic mechanisms for normalizing synaptic serotonin." Medical Hypotheses 65 (1): 138–44. doi:10.1016/j. mehy.2005.01.026. PMID 15893130.

EM Parker and LX Cubeddu (04/01/1988). "Comparative effects of amphetamine, phenylethylamine and related drugs on dopamine efflux, dopamine uptake and mazindol binding." Journal of Pharmacology and Experimental Therapeutics 245 (1): 199–210. ISSN 0022-3565. PMID 3129549.

Medline Plus. "DHEA." Drugs and Supplements Information. National Library of Medicine. Retrieved March 20, 2012.

Medscape (2010). "DHEA Oral." Drug Reference. WebMD LLC. Retrieved March 20, 2012.

The NIH National Library of Medicine — Dehydroepiandrosterone http://www.nlm.nih.gov/medlineplus/druginfo/natural/patient-dhea.html

Selek S, Savas HA, Gergerlioglu HS, et al. The course of nitric oxide and superoxide dismutase during treatment of bipolar depressive episode. J Affect Disord 2008; 107:89-94.

Bilici M, Efe H, Koroglu MA, et al. Antioxidative enzyme activities and lipid peroxidation in major depression: alterations by antidepressant treatments. J Affect Disord 2001; 64:43-51.

Mason R. 200 mg of Zen; L-theanine boosts alpha waves, promotes alert relaxation. Alternative and Complementary Therapies 2001,April; 7:91-95

Chapter 9

Carver JD, Barness LA. Trophic factors for the gastrointestinal tract. Clinical Perinatology 23(2):265-285 (1996). Factors in colostrum which promote the development of the GI tract in newborn infants also help protect against such diseases as Crohn's disease, colitis, necrotizing enterocolitis and diarrhea. PubMed Reference PMID:8780905

Columbia Health Services; Nutritional Value of Carrot Juice; June 4, 2010

University of Maryland Medical Center; Diarrhea; Steven D. Ehrlich, N.M.D.; March 10, 2010.

NYU Langone Medical Center; Low-Fiber/Low-Residue Diet; Maria Adams, M.S., M.PH., R.D.; March 2011.

University of Maryland Medical Center; Crohn's Disease; Steven D. Ehrlich, N.M.D.; Dec. 7, 2008.

MayoClinic.com; Nutrition and Healthy Eating; April 17, 2010.

Rijkers GT, de Vos WM, Brummer RJ, Morelli L, Corthier G, Marteau P; De Vos; Brummer; Morelli; Corthier; Marteau (2011). "Health benefits and health claims of probiotics: Bridging science and marketing." British Journal of Nutrition 106 (9): 1291–6. doi:10.1017/S000711451100287X. PMID 21861940.

"Probiotics in food: health and nutritional properties and guidelines for evaluation." Food and Agricultural Organization of the United Nations and World Health Organization. 1 May 2002.

"Prescription for Herbal Healing"; Phyllis A. Balch; 2002

"Alimentary Pharmacology and Therapeutics"; Randomized, Double-Blind, Placebo-Controlled Trial of Oral Aloe Vera Gel for Active Ulcerative Colitis; L. Langmead, et al.; April 1, 2004.

Chapter 10

Anderson C, French J, Sammons H, Frazer A, Gerrard J, Smellie J (1952). "Coeliac disease; gastrointestinal studies and the effect of dietary wheat flour." Lancet 1 (17): 836–42. doi:10.1016/S0140-6736(52)90795-2. PMID 14918439. doi:10.1136/bmj.2.4900.1318. PMC 2080246. PMID 13209109.

Jensen, Bernard 1987; Chlorella, Gem Of The Oreint; Bernard Jensen, Publisher, Escondido, CA

Zipser R, Farid M, Baisch D, Patel B, Patel D (2005). "Physician awareness of celiac disease: a need for further education." J Gen Intern Med 20 (7): 644–6. doi:10.1007/s11606-005-0111-7. PMC 1490146. PMID 16050861.

Vieth R, et al. Randomized comparison of the effects of vitamin D3 adequate intake versus 100mcg (4000IU) per day on biochemical responses and the wellbeing of patients. Nutrition Journal 2004;3:8

The vitamin D miracle: Is it for real? March 8, 2008 Martin Mittlestaedt

Vieth R(1999). Vitamin D supplementation, 25hydroxyvitamin D concentrations and safety. Am J Clin Nutr 69 (5):842-56. PMID 10232622.

Kim, Young-in, Judith K. Christman 1995; American Journal of Clinical Nutrition; Folate depletion could lower colonic mucosal, vol. 61; 1083-1090

Tierra, Michael 1990; The Way of Herbs; Constipation, 20, 40, 89, 323-324; Simon and Shuster Inc. New York, NY 10020

Fish oil Monograph. Retrieved February 1, 2012, from http//www.hc-sc.gc.ca/ dhp-mps/prodnatur/applications/lilcenprod/momograph/mono_fish_ oil_huile_poisson-eng.php. Natural Health Products Directorate, Health Canada.

A Belluzzi, C Brignola, Mampieri Fish oil and Crohn's disease and Ulcerative colitis: Effect of an enteric-coated fish-oil preparation on relapses in Crohn's disease[PDF] from health4allproducts,com. ...England Journal of ..., 1996 - Mass Medical Soc... The study medications were packed identically and labeled with each patient's code number according to a balanced-block randomization scheme. ... (2005) Postoperative management of ulcerative colitis and Crohn's disease. Current Gastroenterology Reports 7:6, 492-499. 69.

Colter, AL, et al. Fatty acids status and behavioural symptoms of Attention Deficit Hyperactivity Disorder in Adolescents: A case control study. Nutrition Journal, Vol. 7, No. 1, February 14, 2008, (8).

Germanco, M, et al. Plasma, red blood cells phospholipids and clinical evaluation after long chain omega 3 supplementation in children with attention deficit hyperactivity disorder (ADHD). Nutritional Neuroscience, Vol. 10, February, April, 2007. (1-9).

Harris WS, Poston WC, Haddock CK. Tissue n-3 and n-6 fatty acids and risk for coronary artery disease events. Atherosclerosis 2007; 193: 1-10.

Kremer JM. Lawrence DA Petrillo GF. et al. Effects of high dose fish oil on rheumatoid arthritis after stopping nonsteroidal anti inflammatory drugs. Clinical and immune correlates. Arthritis Rheum 1995; 38(8):1107-14.

Chapter 11

Fox, Anthony D. 1993; British Homeopathic Journal; Ulcerative colitis, vol. 82; 179-185.

Chakurski I, Matev M, Koichev A, et al. Treatment of chronic colitis with an herbal combination of Taraxacum officinale,hypericum perforatum, Melissa officinalis, Calendula officinalis, and Foeniculum vulgare. Vutr Boles 1981;20:51-54. (Article in Bulgarian)

Ffcgp, Jack, Ffhom 1990; British Homeopathic Journal; Crohn's Disease, vol. 82; 29-36.

Pizzorno, Joseph E., Michael T. Murray 1996; Textbook Of Natural Medicine; Inflammatory Bowel Disease, vol. 2: VI: InflBD-1-11; Irritable Bowel Syndrome VI: IrrBS-1-3; Bastyr University Publications, Bothell, Washington 98011

Siegel M, Bethune M, Gass J, Ehren J, Xia J, Johannsen A, Stuge T, Gray G, Lee P, Khosla C (2006). "Rational design of combination enzyme therapy for celiac sprue." Chem Biol 13 (6): 649–58. doi:10.1016/j.chembiol.2006.04.009. PMID 16793522.

Hodgson, HJ, Sadler MJ, 1996; International Clinical Nutrition Review; Fish oil; Crohn's Disease, (January), vol.16; 191-192; 179.

J Altern Complement Med.; Artichoke leaf extract ameliorate symptoms of irritable bowel syndrome (IBS) in otherwise healthy volunteers suffering concomitant dyspepsia. 2004 Book pg./5.

Kloss, Jethro 1994; Back To Eden; Colitis, 308-309; Constipation, 237, 309-311; Diverticulosis, 572-573; Back to Eden Books, Publishing Co Loma CA

Lewith, T. George 1995; Complementary Therapies In Medicine; Irritable Bowel Syndrome, vol. 3: 220-223.

Maas H.P.J.A., Arts 1993; British Homeopathic Journal; Ulcerative colitis, vol. 82: 179-185.

Swami Sadashiva Tirtha; The Ayurvedic Encyclopedia, Second Edition, p. 105.

Chapter 12

Haas M.D., Elson; Buck Levin, PhD, RD (2006). Staying Healthy with Nutrition. Berkeley, California: Celestial Arts. ISBN 1-58761-179-1. OCLC 62755545.

"Reports by Single Nutrients." USDA. 2009-02-13. Retrieved 2012-03-19.

U.S. Department of Agriclture, "Labeling Packaged Products," http://www.ams.usda.gov/AMSvl.0/getfile:dDocName=STELDEV3004323&acct=nopgeninfo

Hischenhuber, C; Crevel, R; Jarry, B; Mäki, M; Moneret-Vautrin, D A; Romano, A; Troncone, R; Ward, R (March 2006). "Review article: safe amounts of gluten for patients with wheat allergy or coeliac disease." Aliment. Pharmacol. Ther. 23 (5): 559–75. doi:10.1111/j.1365-2036.2006.02768.x. PMID 16480395.

Tadataka Yamada, Lippincott Williams and Wilkins Green Tea Benefits IBD: Textbook of Gastroenterology, Volume one, 4th edition, 2003 Editor, pages 1141-1142.

Werbach, Melvyn R. 1993: Nutritional Influences on Illness; Constipation, 220-221; Crohn's Disease, 222-226; Irritable Bowel Syndrome, 396-398; Third Line Press, Tarzana, CA

Willett, Walter C., Frank Sacks 1995: American Journal of Clinical Nutrition; Mediterranean diet, vol. 61: 1402S-6S

Bent S, Padula A, Moore D, Patterson M, Mehling W (2006). "Valerian for sleep: a systematic review and meta-analysis." Am. J. Med. 119 (12): 1005–12. doi:10.1016/j.amjmed.2006.02.026. PMID 17145239.

Chapter 13

Rose Elliot: The Bean Book, Fontana/Collins. ISBN 0 00 635536 6

*Safe Gluten-Free Food List (Safe Ingredients) reprinted by permission of www.celiac.com.

ABOUT THE AUTHOR

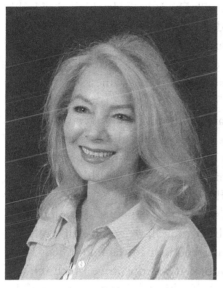

Since my early twenties, my journey has been one of learning the difference that quality nutrition can have on your current state of health and future well-being. While dealing with two health concerns during that time, this journey led me in the direction of vegetable juicing, as I investigated ways to improve my health through diet and supplementation. Because of the many improvements I saw to my general health, and how I simply *felt* different on many levels, I started pursuing career options in this field. I embarked on a two year nutrition-oriented course in Toronto with I.O.N.C. (www.ionc.org). This program included the full scope of education governing the Certified Nutritional Practitioner Designation, the Registered Nutritional Consultant Practitioner Designation and the Registered Orthomolecular Health Practitioner.

Upon completion of this program, it became clear that I would require a university-level education to address widespread medical conditions. I was interested in a traditional degree program that would incorporate mainstream biology, physiology, anatomy while incorporating phyto- and biochemistry, as well as clinical nutrition. My main focus was acquiring enough knowledge to be able to address the causes of disease or conditions, as well as understanding the steps required in the reversal process. It was around this time that I developed an interest in iridology. Through my research, I learned that Westbrook University had the best iridology course available (next to those in England U.K.), along with the course subjects and criteria I was looking for. Eight years later, I received my Doctorate in Holistic Health Sciences. My hard work was rewarded academically when I was presented with an award for Academic Achievement, an honor conferred on students selected from American universities and colleges. Upon obtaining this recognition, I received an invitation to attend Cornell University and a scholarship from Westbrook University.

Within two years of finishing my Ph.D., I opened a Holistic Health Clinic with my husband Ron Honda, called Renew You Holistic Health (www.renewyou.ca) in Ancaster, Ontario, Canada, where I conduct my private practice. A couple of years into my practice, I started lecturing and writing articles for local newspapers and health magazines. I also spent a year as a featured guest at CHML Talk Radio on the Jamie West Show. Occasionally, and upon request, I have spoken to faculty members at Mac Master University on such topics as drug-free pain alternatives and drug and herbal interactions. Other talks have involved women's health, osteoporosis, osteoarthritis, environmental issues, thyroid health, homeopathy, and controlling the pH balance of the body, while ongoing presentations continue to occur locally on various subjects; in particular, gastrointestinal health, hormones, empowering the body to heal, weight loss, and others.

As part of my path, I believe it is important to share knowledge and inspire awareness for non-drug solutions. It was this drive which initially prompted the first edition of this book. To this day, I remain in awe of the body's capacity for rejuvenation and rebalancing when properly supported. It has become one of my life's pleasures to witness how quickly people's symptom complaints fall away, all the while being replaced by renewed expectations for the future.

Visit my website at www.michellehonda.com